Surgical Conditions of the Diaphragm

Guest Editor

GAIL DARLING, MD, FRCSC, FACS

THORACIC SURGERY CLINICS

www.thoracic.theclinics.com

Consulting Editor

MARK K. FERGUSON, MD

November 2009 • Volume 19 • Number 4

SAUNDERS an imprint of ELSEVIER, Inc.

W.B. SAUNDERS COMPANY
A Division of Elsevier Inc.

1600 John F. Kennedy Boulevard • Suite 1800 • Philadelphia, Pennsylvania 19103-2899

http://www.theclinics.com

THORACIC SURGERY CLINICS Volume 19, Number 4
November 2009 ISSN 1547-4127, ISBN-13: 978-1-4377-1392-3, ISBN-10: 1-4377-1392-0

Editor: Catherine Bewick
Developmental Editor: Donald Mumford

Thoracic Surgery Clinics (ISSN 1547-4127) is published quarterly by Elsevier Inc., 360 Park Avenue South, New York, NY 10010-1710. Months of publication are February, May, August, and November. Business and editorial offices: 1600 John F. Kennedy Boulevard, Suite 1800, Philadelphia, PA 19103-2899. Periodicals postage paid at New York, NY, and additional mailing offices. Subscription prices are $242.00 per year (US individuals), $360.00 per year (US institutions), $121.00 per year (US resident/student), $309.00 per year (Canadian individuals), $455.00 per year (Canadian institutions), $165.00 per year (Canadian and foreign students), $329.00 per year (foreign individuals), and $455.00 per year (foreign institutions). Foreign air speed delivery is included in all *Clinics*' subscription prices. All prices are subject to change without notice. **POSTMASTER:** Send address changes to *Thoracic Surgery Clinics*, Elsevier Health Sciences Division, Subscription Customer Service, 3251 Riverport Lane, Maryland Heights, MO 63043. **Customer Service (orders, claims, online, change of address): Telephone: 1-800-654-2452 (U.S. and Canada); 314-447-8871 (outside U.S. and Canada). Fax: 314-447-8029. Email: journalscustomerservice-usa@elsevier.com (for print support); journalsonlinesupport-usa@elsevier.com (for online support).**

Reprints. For copies of 100 or more, of articles in this publication, please contact Commercial Rights Department, Elsevier Inc., 360 Park Avenue South, New York, NY 10010-1710. Tel: (212) 633-3812; Fax: (212) 462-1935; E-mail: reprints@elsevier.com.

Thoracic Surgery Clinics is covered in *MEDLINE/PubMed (Index Medicus)* and *EMBASE/Excerpta Medica.*

Printed and bound by CPI Group (UK) Ltd, Croydon, CR0 4YY

Transferred to Digital Print 2012

Contributors

CONSULTING EDITOR

MARK K. FERGUSON, MD
Professor of Surgery, Section of Cardiac and
Thoracic Surgery, The University of Chicago,
Chicago, Illinois

GUEST EDITOR

GAIL DARLING, MD, FRCSC, FACS
Professor of Surgery, Division of Thoracic
Surgery, Department of Surgery, University of
Toronto; Toronto General Hospital, Toronto,
Ontario, Canada

AUTHORS

NADEEM R. ABU-RUSTUM, MD
Associate Professor, Gynecology Service,
Department of Surgery, Memorial Sloan-
Kettering Cancer Center, New York, New York

RAFAEL S. ANDRADE, MD
Assistant Professor of Surgery, Division of
General Thoracic and Foregut Surgery,
Department of Surgery, University of
Minnesota, Minneapolis, Minnesota

MASAKI ANRAKU, MD
Division of Thoracic Surgery, Toronto General
Hospital, University of Toronto, Toronto,
Ontario, Canada

MAURICE BLITZ, MD, MSc, FRCS(C)
Minimally Invasive Thoracic and Esophageal
Surgery Fellow, Division of Thoracic Surgery,
Swedish Cancer Institute and Medical Center,
Seattle, Washington

DENNIS S. CHI, MD
Associate Member, Gynecology Service,
Department of Surgery, Memorial Sloan-
Kettering Cancer Center, New York,
New York

PRISCILLA P.L. CHIU, MD, PhD
Division of Pediatric General and Thoracic
Surgery, The Hospital for Sick Children,
University of Toronto, Toronto, Ontario,
Canada

GAIL DARLING, MD, FRCSC, FACS
Professor of Surgery, Division of Thoracic
Surgery, Department of Surgery, University of
Toronto; Toronto General Hospital, Toronto,
Ontario, Canada

ANNIE FECTEAU, MD, MHSc, FRCSC
Associate Professor, University of Toronto,
Hospital for Sick Children, Toronto, Ontario,
Canada

**LORENZO E. FERRI, MD, PhD, FRCSC,
FACS**
Assistant Professor of Surgery and Oncology,
Division of Thoracic Surgery, McGill University,
The Montreal General Hospital, Montreal,
Quebec, Canada

DAVID J. FINLEY, MD
Assistant Professor, Thoracic Service,
Department of Surgery, Memorial Sloan-
Kettering Cancer Center, New York, New York

RAJA FLORES, MD
Associate Professor, Thoracic Service, Department of Surgery, Memorial Sloan-Kettering Cancer Center, New York, New York

SEBASTIEN GILBERT, MD
Assistant Professor of Surgery, Division of Thoracic Surgery, Heart, Lung, and Esophageal Surgery Institute, UPMC Presbyterian, Pittsburgh, Pennsylvania

SEAN C. GRONDIN, MD, MPH, FRCSC
Clinical Associate Professor of Surgery, Division of Thoracic Surgery, Foothills Hospital, University of Calgary, Calgary, Alberta, Canada

SHAWN S. GROTH, MD
General Surgery Resident, Department of Surgery, University of Minnesota, Minneapolis, Minnesota

WAËL C. HANNA, MD, MBA
Resident in General Surgery, McGill University, The Montreal General Hospital, Montreal, Quebec, Canada

WAYNE L. HOFSTETTER, MD
Associate Professor, Division of Thoracic and Cardiovascular Surgery, MD Anderson Cancer Center, The University of Texas, Houston, Texas

MIN PETER KIM, MD
Thoracic Surgery Fellow, Division of Thoracic and Cardiovascular Surgery, MD Anderson Cancer Center, The University of Texas, Houston, Texas

MICHAEL AUGUSTINE KO, MD, PhD
Thoracic Surgery Resident, Division of Thoracic Surgery, Department of Surgery, University of Toronto, Toronto General Hospital, Toronto, Ontario, Canada

JACOB C. LANGER, MD
Division of Pediatric General and Thoracic Surgery, The Hospital for Sick Children, University of Toronto, Toronto, Ontario, Canada

BRIAN E. LOUIE, MD, MPH, FRCS(C), FACS
Director, Research and Education and Co-Director, Minimally Invasive Thoracic Surgery Program, Division of Thoracic Surgery, Swedish Cancer Institute and Medical Center, Division of Thoracic Surgery; Seattle, Washington

AHMED NASR, MD, MS (CLIN EPID), FRCSC
Division of Pediatric Surgery, Hospital for Sick Children, Toronto, Ontario, Canada

HEIDI C. ROBERTS, MD
Associate Professor of Radiology, Department of Medical Imaging, University Health Network/Mt Sinai Hospital/Women's College Hospital, Toronto, Ontario, Canada

COLIN SCHIEMAN, MD, FRCSC
Thoracic Surgery Resident, Division of Thoracic Surgery, Foothills Hospital, University of Calgary, Calgary, Alberta, Canada

LANA SCHUMACHER, MD
Cardiothoracic Surgery Resident, Division of Thoracic Surgery, Heart, Lung, and Esophageal Surgery Institute, UPMC Presbyterian, Pittsburgh, Pennsylvania

YARON SHARGALL, MD
Division of Thoracic Surgery, St Joseph Health Centre, University of Toronto, Toronto, Ontario, Canada

Contents

The diaphragm (Greek: dia = in-between, phragma = fence) is a musculoaponeurotic structure that serves as the most important respiratory muscle and the separating structure between the abdominal and thoracic cavities. This article reviews the anatomic components of the diaphragm, its pivotal role in respiration and in the gastroesophageal mechanism, and the surgical implications of the anatomic structuring.

This article describes the normal and abnormal position, motion and morphology of the diaphragm, on chest radiography and fluoroscopy, as well as on computed tomography and magnetic resonance imaging.

Recent advances in the management of congenital diaphragmatic hernia patients have resulted in a dramatic improvement in overall survival. The widespread use of lung-preserving strategies, such as high-frequency oscillatory ventilation and extracorporeal membrane oxygenation, have provided ventilatory or circulatory support for underlying pulmonary hypoplasia while surgical management has been deferred until medical stabilization has occurred. The increased survival, however, has been accompanied by increased neurological, nutritional, and musculoskeletal morbidities among long-term survivors. This article reviews the diagnosis and management strategies of congenital diaphragmatic hernia and the outcomes of congenital diaphragmatic hernia patients.

The article discusses the presentation and treatment of foramen of Morgagni hernia. First, it describes the embryology of the diaphragm along with the incidence of associated anomalies. This is followed by the symptoms, diagnosis, and management. Morgagni hernias are rare and most often asymptomatic; however, there is always a concern about strangulated bowel. Diagnosis is usually by chest radiograph or CT scan. The surgical approach may be either transabdominal or thoracic. Experience is increasing with minimally invasive approaches, which has a low recurrence rate and an excellent prognosis.

Congenital diaphragmatic herniae (CDH) are uncommon in neonates and extremely rare in adults. The clinical presentation of CDH in adults tends to be very different from neonates. Many adults remain asymptomatic and CDH are diagnosed incidentally. All CDH should be repaired. Minimally invasive surgical approaches are now gaining popularity for the repair of CDH with excellent outcomes.

Few topics within thoracic surgery are as controversial as the management of paraesophageal hernias (PEH). In this article, the types of hiatal hernia are classified and the clinical presentation and evaluation of patients with PEH are discussed. Controversies in the management of PEH including the indications for surgery, the different operative approaches, and the role of esophageal shortening are reviewed. Finally, the evidence regarding the need for fundoplication or fixation of the stomach with gastropexy or gastrostomy and the use of prosthetic material in performing the hiatal closure are examined.

Acute diaphragmatic hernia is a result of diaphragmatic injury that accompanies severe blunt or penetrating thoracoabdominal trauma. The incidence, characteristics, and diagnosis of acute diaphragmatic hernia are discussed. Acute traumatic diaphragmatic injuries are treated by surgical reduction of the herniated organs, if present, and closure of the diaphragmatic defect. The various treatment options are discussed. Outcomes of acute diaphragmatic hernia repair are largely dictated by the severity of concomitant injuries, with the Injury Severity Score being the most widely recognized predictor of mortality.

Traumatic diaphragmatic hernia encompasses a spectrum of disease ranging from acute to chronic. Chronic traumatic diaphragmatic hernia is uncommon and associated with significant morbidity and mortality. Multiplanar CT with coronal, sagittal, and axial reconstructions is most effective in making this diagnosis. Once diagnosed, repair should be undertaken. Open transthoracic repair is preferred. Basic hernia repair principles apply including the construction of a tension-free repair, which may necessitate the use of prosthetics.

Acquired diaphragmatic paralysis is an uncommon cause of respiratory insufficiency in adults. Symptoms of diaphragmatic paralysis range in severity from mild alterations in exercise capacity to severe, life-threatening illness. For well-selected patients, diaphragmatic plication is indicated for symptomatic relief. Plication may be performed via standard thoracotomy or by video-assisted techniques.

Diaphragmatic Eventration

Shawn S. Groth and Rafael S. Andrade

Diaphragmatic eventration is defined as thinning of the diaphragm secondary to a congenital deficiency in diaphragmatic muscle structure. Clinically, diaphragmatic eventration can be impossible to differentiate from acquired paralysis. Diaphragmatic plication is indicated for symptomatic patients and leads to significant improvement in symptoms, quality of life, and pulmonary function tests.

Tumors of the Diaphragm

Min Peter Kim and Wayne L. Hofstetter

Primary tumors of the diaphragm are very rare. Benign tumors of the diaphragm are resected if symptomatic or if there is concern for malignancy. Malignant tumors are either primary, metastatic, or the result of direct extension to the diaphragm from adjacent malignancy. Malignant tumors are treated based on histology and response to chemotherapy, with surgical resection performed when feasible.

Reconstructive Techniques After Diaphragm Resection

David J. Finley, Nadeem R. Abu-Rustum, Dennis S. Chi, and Raja Flores

Diaphragm resection requires complete reconstruction to avoid respiratory compromise or herniation of abdominal contents into the chest. Primary reconstruction of the diaphragm is often possible, even with a large defect, as long as the tissue can come together without excessive tension. Larger defects or complete diaphragm resections necessitate reconstruction with synthetic material or autologous tissue. These reconstructions can be accomplished safely and effectively by following specific surgical tenets, and require an in-depth knowledge of the diaphragm's anatomy, innervation, blood supply, and adjacent organs.

Index

Thoracic Surgery Clinics

THE CLINICS ARE NOW AVAILABLE ONLINE!

Access your subscription at:
www.theclinics.com

Preface

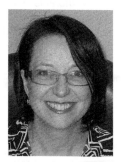

Gail Darling, MD, FRCSC, FACS
Guest Editor

The integrity and function of the diaphragm is essential to life because of its role in respiration. It is similar to the heart in that the muscle of the diaphragm must contract continuously throughout life. Any breach or dysfunction of the diaphragm may be a threat to life; hence, a thorough knowledge of the anatomy, physiology, and conditions of the diaphragm are essential to the practice of thoracic surgery. Thoracic surgeons must be able to repair or reconstruct the diaphragm when its integrity is breached by congenital abnormalities, acquired hernias, trauma, tumors, or surgical incisions. In acquired conditions that diminish diaphragmatic function, thoracic surgeons may be required to surgically modify the diaphragm to improve function. Knowledge of the innervation of the diaphragm allows surgeons to plan incisions in the diaphragm to minimize dysfunction. The diaphragm also has an important function in gastrointestinal function in esophageal emptying and emesis and as an antireflux barrier.

This edition of the *Thoracic Surgery Clinics* addresses the anatomy and physiology, imaging modalities, congenital and acquired hernias, traumatic injuries, eventration and paralysis, tumors, and reconstructive techniques that form the basis for thoracic surgery of the diaphragm. Drs Shargall and Anraku, from St Joseph's Health Sciences Centre in Toronto, Canada, have addressed the anatomy and physiology relevant to surgeons. Imaging the diaphragm has historically been challenging but modern techniques, including MRI, as comprehensively reviewed by Dr Heidi Roberts from the University Health Network in Toronto,

Canada, provides surgeons with clear diagnostic imaging on which to base a surgical plan.

Diagnosis and management of congenital diaphragmatic hernias has evolved significantly with advances in prenatal imaging and understanding of the pulmonary pathophysiology, particularly associated with posterior congenital diaphragmatic hernia. Posterior congenital hernias are thoroughly reviewed by Drs Chiu and Langer from the Hospital for Sick Children in Toronto, Canada, and anterior congenital hernias are reviewed by Drs Nasr and Fecteau from the same institution.

Diaphragmatic hernias in adults include congenital diaphragmatic hernias that do not become apparent until later in life. Drs Schumacher and Gilbert from the University of Pittsburgh Medical Center in Pittsburgh, Pennsylvania, provide a clear review of the diagnosis and management of these hernias. Similarly, traumatic diaphragmatic hernias may present acutely or may be occult and present years after the initiating event. Acute traumatic diaphragmatic hernias are thoroughly addressed by Drs Hanna and Ferri from McGill University in Montreal, Canada, and chronic traumatic hernia is discussed by Drs Blitz and Louie from the Swedish Medical Center, Seattle, Washington. Paraesophageal hernias are a challenging problem and controversy exists as to the best approach to these complex problems. Drs Scheimann and Grondin from the University of Calgary, Alberta, Canada, have provided a comprehensive review of the issues. Impaired diaphragmatic function may result from acquired paralysis or, less

Thorac Surg Clin 19 (2009) ix–x
doi:10.1016/j.thorsurg.2009.08.012

commonly, eventration. Dr Ko and I address the diagnosis and management of acquired paralysis, and eventration and its management are reviewed by Dr Andrade from the University of Minnesota.

Tumors of the diaphragm are rare but the diaphragm not infrequently is secondarily involved, usually by direct invasion. The approach to such tumors is comprehensively presented by Drs Min and Hofstetter from the MD Anderson Cancer Center in Houston, Texas. Reconstructive techniques are an essential part of every thoracic surgeon's armamentarium and these are clearly presented by Dr Flores from the Memorial Sloan–Kettering Cancer Center in New York.

I wish to thank the contributing authors for their excellent work. This edition of the *Thoracic Surgery Clinics*, entitled "Surgical Conditions of the Diaphragm," provides thoracic surgery trainees and practicing thoracic surgeons with a comprehensive and practical review that they can use in everyday practice.

Gail Darling, MD, FRCSC, FACS
Division of Thoracic Surgery
Department of Surgery
University of Toronto
Toronto General Hospital, 9N-955
200 Elizabeth Street
Toronto, Canada, ON M5G 2C4

E-mail address:
gail.darling@uhn.on.ca

Surgical Conditions of the Diaphragm: Anatomy and Physiology

Masaki Anraku, MD[a], Yaron Shargall, MD[b],*

KEYWORDS

- Diaphragm • Anatomy • Physiology • Surgery
- Surgical incisions

The diaphragm (Greek: dia = in-between, phragma = fence) is a musculoaponeurotic structure that serves as the most important respiratory muscle and the separating structure between the abdominal and thoracic cavities. This article reviews the anatomic components of the diaphragm, its pivotal role in respiration and in the gastroesophageal mechanism, and the surgical implications of the anatomic structuring.

ANATOMY

In adults, the diaphragm represents less than 0.5% of body weight,[1] but it is the most important muscle in the human body after the heart (**Box 1**). It is composed of a central noncontractile tendon and two major muscular portions: the costal and crural diaphragm. An additional minor muscular portion is the sternal part of the diaphragm. The diaphragm is an elliptical cylindroid structure, capped by a dome[2]; it arches over the abdomen, with the right hemidiaphragm higher than the left. The concave, dome-shaped part allows the liver and the spleen, situated underneath the diaphragm, to be protected by the lower ribs and the chest wall. The caudal and cranial views of the diaphragm with the various anatomic structures are shown in **Figs. 1** and **2**.

Embryology

The diaphragm is formed by four embryologic entities, including (1) the septum transversum, (2) the pleuroperitoneal membranes, (3) the dorsal mesentery of esophagus, and (4) the body wall muscles.[3]

The septum transversum is derived from mesoderm and this structure forms the central tendon of the diaphragm, a process that starts during the third embryonic week. Between this week and the eighth week, the developing diaphragm descends from the level of C3 to the final position at the level of L1, carrying with it the phrenic nerves, which originate from the third to fifth cervical levels. Right and left sides of pleuroperitoneal membranes attach to the septum transversum laterally and caudally and to the dorsal mesentery medially. The right and left pleuroperitoneal membranes ultimately close at approximately the eighth week of gestation and separate the thoracic and abdominal cavities. The dorsal mesentery of the esophagus attaches the foregut to the dorsal body wall and eventually becomes the crura of the diaphragm. The pleural cavities and their costodiaphragmatic recesses split the inner and outer layers of the body wall between the 9th and 12th weeks of gestations; the inner layer of the body wall muscle composes the posterolateral portion of the diaphragm, and the outer layer of the body wall becomes the thoracic wall.

The costal part of the diaphragm develops from the lateral body walls whereas the crural part of the diaphragm originates from the dorsal mesentery of the esophagus, which explains why the diaphragm is characterized by two separate functional components, the costal diaphragm and the crural diaphragm.[4,5]

[a] Division of Thoracic Surgery, Toronto General Hospital, University of Toronto, 200 Elizabeth Street, Toronto, Ontario M5G2C4, Canada
[b] Division of Thoracic Surgery, St Joseph Health Centre, University of Toronto, 30 The Queensway, SSW W221, Toronto, Ontario M6R 1B5, Canada
* Corresponding author.
E-mail address: shargy@stjoe.on.ca (Y. Shargall).

Thorac Surg Clin 19 (2009) 419–429
doi:10.1016/j.thorsurg.2009.08.002
1547-4127/09/$ – see front matter © 2009 Elsevier Inc. All rights reserved.

Box 1
Anatomy

- The diaphragm is composed of a central non-contractile tendon and two major muscular portions: the costal and crural diaphragm.

- The costal and crural parts of diaphragm have different embryologic origins, different segmental innervation, and different functional properties.

- Major blood supply is from the pericardiophrenic, musculophrenic (from the internal thoracic artery), superior phrenic (from the thoracic aorta), and inferior phrenic (from the abdominal aorta) arteries.

- From the surgical perspective, understanding the phrenic nerve distribution on the diaphragm is of crucial importance to avoid injury to the nerve during diaphragmatic incisions.

The Muscular Parts of the Diaphragm

The diaphragm is a striated skeletal muscle consisting of two major parts: the muscular part radiating outward and the central, noncontractile tendinous part. The muscular part of the diaphragm has three components, which originate from the lumbar spine dorsally, ribs laterally, and sternum ventrally. The three muscular components are separated from each other by muscle-free gaps and are named (1) the lumbar (pars lumbaris), (2) costal (pars costalis), and (3) sternal (pars sternalis) parts. The muscle fibers of the lumber (crural) diaphragm project onto the antero-lateral aspect of L1 to L3 whereas those of the costal diaphragm project from the central tendon to the upper margins of the lower 6 ribs and the xiphoid process of the sternum.

Lumbar (crural) part (pars lumbalis)

The lumbar (crural) part of the diaphragm forms the right and left crura along the lumbar spine. It is the most powerful part of the diaphragm. The right crus arises from the anterior surface of lumbar vertebrae (L1-4 on the right and L1-2 on the left), the intervertebral disks, and the anterior longitudinal ligament. The right crus is larger than the left crus, and it directs to the middle part of the central tendon on both sides of the medial plane superiorly. The right crus splits to form the esophageal hiatus in more than 60% of individuals (whereas in the rest, the esophageal crura is derived by contribution of both crurae), functioning as a sphincter-like opening of the diaphragm (the

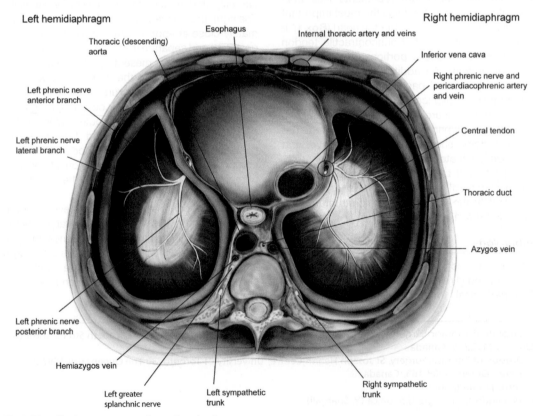

Left hemidiaphragm

Esophagus

Thoracic (descending) aorta

Internal thoracic artery and veins

Right hemidiaphragm

Inferior vena cava

Left phrenic nerve anterior branch

Right phrenic nerve and pericardiacophrenic artery and vein

Left phrenic nerve lateral branch

Central tendon

Thoracic duct

Azygos vein

Left phrenic nerve posterior branch

Hemiazygos vein

Left greater splanchnic nerve

Left sympathetic trunk

Right sympathetic trunk

Fig. 1. The diaphragm as seen from the chest.

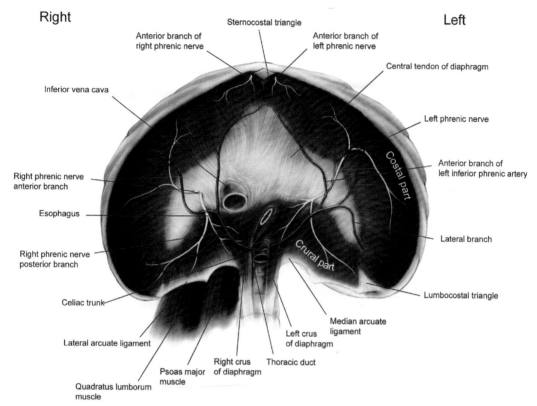

Fig. 2. The diaphragm as seen from the abdomen.

esophageal hiatus), and the split muscle fibers meet again to form the anterior margin of the aortic opening. Although the esophageal crura consists of muscular and tendinous tissues, only the tendinous part is strong enough to hold sutures during surgery. In 90% of patients, however, the medial edge of the crura is tendinous, allowing for a safe suturing.[6] Inferiorly, the right crus forms the ligament of Treitz, a portion of the suspensory muscle of the duodenum, which runs downward to the left of the celiac artery. The left crus, alternatively, directs upward to the left of the esophageal hiatus. It is much smaller than the right crus. A separate part of the left crus reaches to the central tendon, running behind the muscle fibers of the right crus.

Costal part (pars costalis)

The costal part of the diaphragm originates from the inner surface and upper margins of the six lower (caudal) ribs and radiates into the central tendon. The lumbocostal triangles/trigones (Bochdalek's gap) exist between the lumbar and costal parts of the diaphragm, more commonly on the left side than on the right side. In these areas, the gaps are usually closed only by fascia, peritoneum, and pleura. Anteriorly, there are bilateral

triangular gaps between the sternal and costal parts of the diaphragm (discussed later).

Sternal part

The sternal part of the diaphragm originates with small dentations from the posterior layer of the rectus sheath and from the back of the xiphoid process, inserting at the central tendon (see **Fig. 2**). Lateral to it (on both sides), there is a narrow gap between the sternal and costal parts, which is usually composed of connective tissue only. These gaps (named after Morgagni and Larrey, or the sternocostal triangles) pass the internal thoracic/superior epigastric vessels and are potential sources for herniation, more commonly seen in adults (**Fig. 3**).

Tendinous Part of the Diaphragm (Central Tendon)

Essentially, all the musculature of the diaphragm inserts on the thickened central tendon, which is the highest part of the diaphragm. The tendinous part is a fascial aponeurosis that has a cloverleaf-like shape consisting of three leaflets (one anterior and two lateral leaves) separated from each other by slight indentations. In contrast to its name, the central tendon is not located

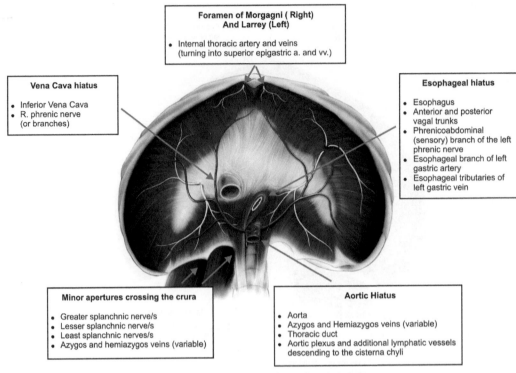

**Foramen of Morgagni (Right)
And Larrey (Left)**

- Internal thoracic artery and veins
  (turning into superior epigastric a. and vv.)

Vena Cava hiatus

- Inferior Vena Cava
- R. phrenic nerve
  (or branches)

Esophageal hiatus

- Esophagus
- Anterior and posterior
  vagal trunks
- Phrenicoabdominal
  (sensory) branch of the left
  phrenic nerve
- Esophageal branch of left
  gastric artery
- Esophageal tributaries of
  left gastric vein

Minor apertures crossing the crura

- Greater splanchnic nerve/s
- Lesser splanchnic nerve/s
- Least splanchnic nerves/s
- Azygos and hemiazygos veins (variable)

Aortic Hiatus

- Aorta
- Azygos and Hemiazygos veins (variable)
- Thoracic duct
- Aortic plexus and additional lymphatic vessels
  descending to the cisterna chyli

Fig. 3. Structures passing through the diaphragm, as seen from the abdomen.

centrally, and it is not symmetric. It lies more anteriorly than posteriorly (with the posterior crural muscular fibers longer than the anterior ones), and the right leaf of the tendon is the largest of all three. A midanterior portion extends toward the xiphoid process of the sternum, and other portions radiate posterolaterally, the left leaflet a little narrower than the right one. The central portion of the tendon is located underneath the pericardium, thus the superior surface of the

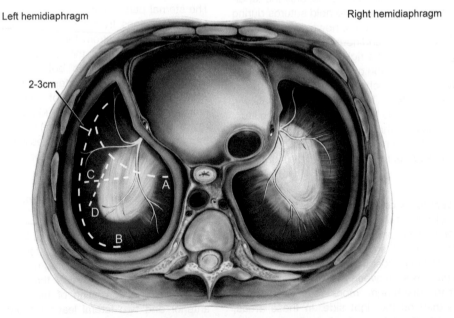

Left hemidiaphragm

Right hemidiaphragm

2-3cm

Fig. 4. Surgical incisions on the diaphragm. (*A*) An incision with a risk of total paralysis of the diaphragm. (*B*) A preferred incision with minimal risk of nerve injury. (*C, D*) Incisions in safe areas, but with small risk of nerve injury.

tendinous part is attached firmly to the pericardium. Lateral to the heart, the right and left diaphragmatic dome parts are mobile, and their position is dependent on the extent of ventilation. At resting position, the right dome is at the level of the fourth intercostal space, whereas the left dome is at the fifth intercostal space. In deep inspirium, both domes descend approximately two intercostal levels lower than their resting position. The foramen of the inferior vena cava is located in the tendinous part of the diaphragm to the right of the midline.

Blood Supply of the Diaphragm

The diaphragm has an enormously rich blood supply. As a result, necrosis of the diaphragm is extremely rare. The arterial blood supply to the diaphragm is derived from (1) the pericardiophrenic arteries, (2) the musculophrenic arteries, (3) the superior and inferior phrenic arteries, and (4) the intercostal arteries. The pericardiophrenic arteries run through the chest along with the phrenic nerves, then distribute on the thoracic side of the diaphragm. The musculophrenic arteries (branched from the internal thoracic arteries) and the superior phrenic arteries (branched from the thoracic aorta) also provide blood supply to the thoracic side of the diaphragm. The right and left internal thoracic arteries pass through the Morgagni's (right) and Larrey's (left) gaps after giving rise to the musculophrenic arteries, and then become the superior epigastric arteries.

The right and left inferior phrenic arteries, direct branches from the abdominal aorta or from the celiac trunk, supply the abdominal side of the diaphragm. They are much larger than the other arterial branches and are the main source for arterial blood supply to the diaphragm. On rare occasions, the right renal artery gives rise to the right inferior phrenic artery. The peripheral parts of the costal diaphragm have an additional blood supply from the intercostal arteries. These arteries form anastomoses with the superior and inferior phrenic arteries to maintain blood flow to the diaphragm.[7]

The veins of the diaphragm follow the arteries. The venous drainage from the thoracic side of the diaphragm is via the azygos and hemiazygos systems, whereas that of the abdominal side is mainly via the inferior phrenic veins to the inferior vena cava. Venous drainage of the peripheral costal and sternal portions of the diaphragm is via the intercostal and the internal thoracic veins, respectively. These vessels are accompanied by lymphatic vessels.

The diaphragmatic blood flow is respiratory-phase dependent: it increases during the diaphragmatic relaxation (resting) phase, decreases during inspiration phase, and can be completely diminished during forceful inspiration.[7] Resistive loading ventilation increases blood flow to the diaphragm much more than unobstructed ventilation. Animal studies showed that during resistance breathing, diaphragmatic blood flow increased 26-fold, whereas the blood flow to the rest of the inspiratory and expiratory muscles increased to a lesser extent.[8] Increased intramuscular pressure during muscle contraction attributes to blood flow restriction.[9] Because the diaphragmatic contractility is dependent on the blood circulation with an appropriate oxygen supply, it is important that the diaphragm returns to its constant resting position with optimal relaxation, which allows for diaphragmatic blood flow to occur. Another mechanical factor influencing the diaphragmatic blood flow is the change in the intrathoracic and intra-abdominal pressures. Increased intra-abdominal pressure produced by diaphragmatic contraction leads to blood flow limitation.[10] Hypoxemia increases blood flow to the diaphragm, an adaptive mechanism in patients with chronic obstructive pulmonary disease (COPD), in whom faster respiratory rate and smaller tidal volumes might help to preserve diaphragmatic performance.[11]

Lymphatic System of the Diaphragm

The thoracic and abdominal surfaces of the diaphragm have a rich lymphatic system accompanying the blood vessels. The lymphatic vessels from the abdominal side of the diaphragm are distributed parallel to the blood vessels. The anterior (ventral) lymphatic system drains to the parasternal nodes. Right and left lateral lymphatic systems run along with the phrenic nerves. Their efferent lymphatics drain into the lymph nodes of the posterior mediastinum (brachiocephalic and parasternal nodes). The posterior (dorsal) lymphatic vessels drain to the lateral aortic and posterior mediastinal lymph nodes. The diaphragmatic lymphatic drainage system plays a major role in the absorption of material from the peritoneal cavity.

Innervation of the Diaphragm

Motor and sensory innervations are supplied by the phrenic nerve and the sixth or seventh intercostal nerves, the latter distributed to the costal part of the diaphragm. The muscular part of the diaphragm receives its main motor innervation via the phrenic nerve. The right and left phrenic nerves originate in the cervical plexus (mainly the fourth cervical nerve roots, with lesser contributions from the third and fifth roots) and run craniocaudally toward the diaphragm, passing anterior to the hilum of the lungs, attaching to the pericardium along with the pericardiophrenic artery and veins where they provide pericardial branches. The right phrenic nerve descends along the superior vena cava, subsequently along the side of the pericardium anterior to the right pulmonary hilum, then enters into the central tendon anterolaterally to the vena caval opening. The left phrenic nerve descends laterally to the side of the aortic arch and runs downward along the side of the pericardium, anterior to the left pulmonary hilum. Thereafter, it enters into the diaphragm lateral to the left border of the heart and anterior to the central tendon. The phrenic nerves give branches on the thoracic side of the diaphragm. Once the right and left phenic nerves pass through the diaphragm, they branch off anteromedially to the sternum, anterolaterally to the costal diaphragm, and posteromedially to the crural diaphragm. The left phrenic nerve also passes through the esophageal hiatus to the peritoneum and several upper abdominal organs. These diaphragmatic branches are not always visible directly even after removal of the diaphragmatic pleura because the branches extend into the muscle of the diaphragm.

Understanding the distribution of the phrenic nerves on the diaphragm is of significant importance if diaphragmatic incision is considered during surgery (eg, left thoracoabdominal incision) because phrenic nerve injury could cause significant loss of diaphragmatic function. Surgical incisions can generally be safely made without injury to the phrenic nerves because the anatomic arrangement of the nerve branches is constant in most cases. The diaphragmatic branches of the phrenic nerves, however, are commonly embedded deep in the muscle and are not exposed on the undersurface of the diaphragm. Therefore, one cannot rely on visualization of those branches before incising the diaphragm (**Fig. 4**).

Openings in the Diaphragm

The diaphragm has three anatomic openings: the aortic, the esophageal, and the inferior vena cava orifices. Other small openings include a triangular gap between the sternal and costal parts of the diaphragm bilaterally and between the costal and lateral arcuate ligaments bilaterally, respectively (see **Fig. 3**).

The aortic hiatus is located anterior to the lower border of T12 or L1 and is bordered dorsally by the

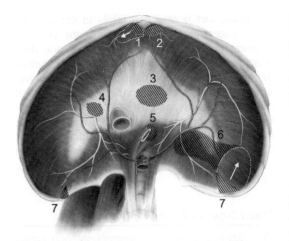

Fig. 5. Potential diaphragmatic defects/hernias. **1.** Morgagni's. **2.** Larrey's. **3.** Peritoneopericardial communication (defect of the septum transversum). **4.** Paracaval hernia. **5.** Hiatal hernia. **6.** Pleuroperitoneal (see **Fig. 6**). **7.** Bochdalek's (lumbocostal triangle/ trigone). Both short and long *arrows* indicate direction of potential extension.

vertebral body, laterally by the crural diaphragm, and ventrally by the median arcuate ligaments. This hiatus transmits the aorta, the aortic plexus, the thoracic duct, lymphatic vessels that descend from the thorax to the cisterna chili,[2] and (usually) the azygos vein. The median arcuate ligament forms a tendinous arch in front of the aortic hiatus at the level of the celiac trunk and connects the two cruras of the diaphragm. It may be used for surgical narrowing and reconstruction of the esophageal hiatus.[3] Incidental injury to the thoracic duct during manipulations of the aorta along the hiatus might result in chylous ascites and occasionally result in chylothorax due to injury higher into the chest or chyle leakage from the abdominal side of the hiatus into the pleural cavity.

The esophageal hiatus is an oval aperture located at the level of T10 on the left of the midline and ventrally to the aortic hiatus behind the central tendon. It is formed by the diaphragmatic crura anterolaterally by splitting of the medial fibers of the right crus and posteriorly by the median arcuate ligament. Ventrally, this hiatus is framed by muscle fibers. As a result of this anatomic structuring, diaphragmatic contraction can contribute to the closure of the caudal end of the esophagus. The esophageal hiatus transmits the esophagus, the anterior and posterior vagal nerve trunks, and the phrenicoabdominal (sensory) branch of the left phrenic nerve (eventually supplying the pancreas and peritoneum). The phrenoesophageal ligament, the fascia on the inferior surface of the diaphragm extending to the esophageal wall approximately 2 cm above the gastroesophageal junction, limits the upward displacement of the esophagus. Other structures passing through this hiatus include esophageal branches and tributaries of the left gastric artery and vein.

The foramen vena cava is located at the right portion of the central tendon at the level of T8 and T9, thus its margins are tendinous. The right phrenic nerve also passes through this foramen and few lymphatics.[12] Although a source for controversy for years, it is believed that the vena caval blood flow to the heart is facilitated by ventilation as the foramen vena cava is stretched by the diaphragmatic contraction during inspiration.[6]

The internal thoracic artery and veins extend down through the Larrey's and Morgagni's gaps (left and right, respectively [see **Fig. 3**]) and from then on are termed the superior epigastric artery and veins, respectively. Few lymphatics usually accompany those vessels through the gaps. Morgagni's hernia (see 'Congenital Hernia in Adults') are more common on the right gap because the left is protected by the pericardium. Given the relationship with the peritoneum, most hernias contain a sac, and the most commonly herniating structures are the colon and the omentum.

Posteriorly, the lumbocostal triangle between the costal portion of the diaphragm and the portion arising from the lateral arcuate ligament (bilaterally but mostly on the left side) might contain only few muscle fibers, and only pleura and peritoneum divide the abdominal and thoracic cavities. This defect, the foramen of Bochdalek, might extend further anteriorly and medially and is the site of congenital diaphragmatic hernia or, rarely, similar hernia in adults. Additional potential openings/ defects in the diaphragm, such as peritoneopericardial hernia, paracaval, and pleuroperitoneal hernias (see **Fig. 5**), are extremely rare. They have been described in newborns and are rarely seen in adults in association with trauma (**Fig. 6**); in late presentation of diaphragmatic tear through a potential pleuroperitoneal defect; and in asymptomatic patients with an incidental finding of left pleuroperitoneal hernia (**Fig. 7**). Other structures passing between the thorax and the abdomen, through the diaphragm or posterior to it, are shown in **Fig. 3**. Those include the splanchnic nerves and occasionally the azygos or hemiazygos veins.

Diaphragmatic Pores

Passage of fluids, gases, or tissues transdiaphragmatically through pores in the diaphragm was recognized but not well defined until comprehensively reviewed by Kirchner in 1998.[13] Diaphragmatic pores/holes might be single or multiple, ranging in

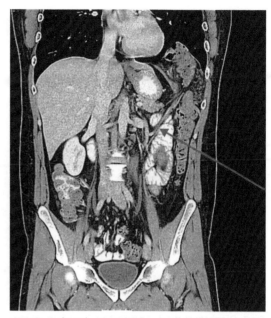

Fig. 6. Delayed traumatic diaphragmatic hernia through a potential pleuroperitoneal defect in a 25 year old, presenting with bowel obstruction 2 years after blunt trauma. Notice the stretched venous branch of the superior mesenteric vein passing through the defect (*arrow*), suggesting chronic process.

size from a tiny pinhole to up to a centimeter, and are usually located in the tendinous part of the diaphragm, most commonly on the right side. The majority of defects are believed acquired. Although the precise mechanism is unknown, the transdiaphragmatic pressure gradient between the peritoneal and pleural cavities premotes transfer from the abdomen to the thorax. The acquired pores are a result of a challenge to the diaphragmatic integrity by various space-occupying materials that increase the intra-abdominal pressure. Although the so-called porous diaphragm syndrome[13] has many causes, the common clinical presentation is that of thoracic symptoms and signs (pleural effusion, hemothorax, empyema, pneumothorax) secondary to the abdominal pathology. The most common manifestations are cirrhotic hydrothorax, secondary to ascites, and iatrogenic ascites with hydrothorax secondary to peritoneal dialysis. Another clinically significant scenario is tension pneumothorax during laparoscopic surgery. The role of diaphragmatic pores in catamenial pneumothorax is not completely defined, although diaphragmatic pores are found in large proportions of cases.

When found, (thoracoscopic) closure of pores is curative in patients with ascitic or peritoneal dialysis induced hydrothorax. In many patients, the

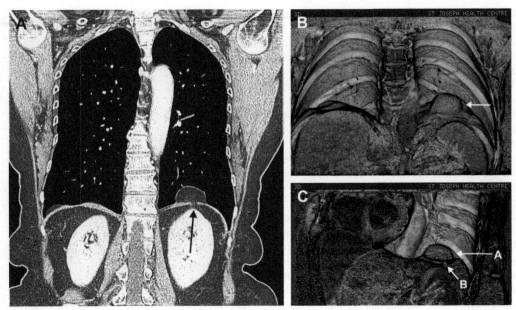

Fig. 7. Diaphragmatic 3-D reconstruction of an asymptomatic 72-year-old woman investigated for "lung mass" on a yearly chest readiograph. There was no previous history of trauma. (*A, B*) A posterior defect of the left hemidiaphragm is clearly seen (*arrow*). (*C*) The defect can be defined as peluroperitoneal type hernia (*arrow A*), containing omental fat (*arrow B*).

diaphragm might be found intact during thoracoscopy. Pleurodesis should always be considered.

Anatomical Consideration in Surgery

Diaphragmatic incisions are necessary for various thoracic or abdominal procedures. They should be carefully made to avoid significant injury to major branches of the phrenic nerve and important vascular structures (in particular, the right and left inferior phrenic arteries). Due to the rapid decrease in size of the phrenic nerve branches and their positioning embedded in the muscle, it is not practical to try and follow them. The radial incision (see **Fig. 4**A) from the costal margin to the esophageal hiatus was used in the past, but resulted in complete paralysis of the hemidiaphragm and is now abandoned. Incisions in various safe areas can be carried with little risk for phrenic nerve damage (see **Fig. 4**C, D) but are not optimal due to a limited surgical exposure. Although incisions made into the central tendon rarely cause diaphragmatic paralysis (phrenic nerve distribution [see **Fig. 4**]), they also provide only minimal exposure of the abdomen. The safety of cutting through the central tendon can be useful during repair of traumatic diaphragmatic tears and various acquired diaphragmatic hernias, where the opening in the diaphragm is often small, and an enlargement is frequently required to

allow for a safe reduction of abdominal contents back into the peritoneal cavity. Transdiaphragmatic exposure of the cardia can be achieved using a septum transversum incision from the anterior portion of the esophageal hiatus anterolaterally but it risks injury to the left phrenic nerve and is not commonly used. The most commonly used incision is the circumferential incision at the periphery of the diaphragm. It allows for an excellent exposure of the abdominal contents from the chest and vice versa, with minimal risk for nerve injury (see **Fig. 4**B). Using a cautery, a diaphragmatic rim of 2 to 3 cm parallel to the chest wall should be maintained, as a smaller rim makes closure technically demanding, and marking sutures should be placed to ensure correct orientation of the edges upon closure. It is generally easier to start the incision anteriorly, lateral to the pericardium, and carry it circumferentially as far posteriorly as needed, using the anterolateral two thirds for procedures associated with antireflux repairs, and more posterior extension (when needed) for esophageal resections. Used on the left side, this incision usually encounters the main branch of the inferior phrenic artery, requiring division and ligation of the vessel. When thoracoabdominal approach is selected, this incision can be extended and started medially between the pericardial attachment to the diaphragm and the entrance of the phrenic nerve into the diaphragm.

PHYSIOLOGY

The diaphragm has two major physiologic functions: (1) to support respiration and (2) to support gastroesophageal functions, including esophageal emptying, antireflux barrier, and emesis. The costal part of the diaphragm supports mainly respiration (especially during inspiration), whereas the crural part of the diaphragm has an important role in gastrointestinal function. The diaphragm gives additional powers to any expulsive acts; a deep inspiration is taken place before sneezing, coughing, laughing, crying, and before the expulsion of urine or feces. The diaphragm also provides anatomic stability to thoracic and abdominal organs.

The Role of the Diaphragm in Respiration

The diaphragm is the most important respiratory muscle, responsible for the majority of the work of breathing in normal individuals and those with lung diseases (**Box 2**). Paralysis of all nondiaphragmatic respiratory muscles usually does not result in respiratory failure, whereas bilateral diaphragmatic paralysis usually causes carbon dioxide retention and respiratory failure.[2] The inspiratory mechanism of the diaphragm is a combination of three pathways, all of which are significantly influenced by the cranial-caudal orientation of the muscle fibers and the existence of the zone of opposition (the area of contact between the diaphragm and the rib cage) First, as the muscle fibers shorten, they pull the central tendon in a caudal direction, thus expanding chest volumes with a piston-like action. At the same time of inspiration, the dome of the diaphragm descends, thus pushing the abdominal organs down and increasing the intra-abdominal pressure. This elevated pressure is transmitted across the apposition zone, pushing the lower ribs outward, resulting in expansion of the rib cage.

Box 2
The diaphragm in respiratory function

- The costal part of the diaphragm is the major muscle for inspiration and is composed of type I, slow-twitch, fatigue-resistant muscle fibers and type II, fast-twitch, fatiguing muscle fibers.

- A fiber-type shift from type II to type I occurs to adapt to a chronic changes in obstructive pulmonary disease.

- Diffuse atrophy of the costal diaphragm is seen in patients who undergo prolonged ventilation with diaphragmatic inactivity.

Finally, the relationship of the contracting, descending diaphragm to the opposing effect of the abdominal contents serves as a fulcrum. The net effect is force exerted on the lower ribs cranially, resulting in their upward and outward movement.[14]

The costal part of the diaphragm is the main musculature for the act of respiration, specifically the inspiratory phase. Breathing is endurance work, like that of the heart, as the diaphragm must contract in repetitive fashion for life. The muscle fibers of the diaphragm are well suited for this task; up to 55% of the fibers in adult human diaphragm are type I, slow-twitch, which are highly resistant to fatigue.[15] The remaining muscle fibers are type II, fast-twitch that are susceptible to fatigue. Type II fibers are 21% IIA, rapid oxidative fibers and 24% IIB, rapid glycolytic fibers.[16] In normal breathing, type I muscle fibers are mainly used. Fast-twitch type II muscle fibers are recruited when the breathing rate increases because the fundamental contractile unit in muscle is more in type II than in type I fibers.[17]

The shape of the diaphragm is an elliptical cylinder capped by a dome.[14] This unique shape gives the ability to increase the dimensions of the chest cavity to inflate the lungs. In resting position, the diaphragm forms a dome concave toward the abdomen in right and left sides. The diaphragmatic muscle is active during inspiration; its contraction causes descent of the diaphragm that results in outward movement of the abdominal wall.[2] The dome of the diaphragm in each side moves downward nearly parallel to its original position during deep inspiration. This increased diaphragmatic tension produces a caudally oriented force onto the central tendon and a cephalically oriented force onto ribs 7 to 12 (costal part) and the vertebral column (crural part). The caudally and cephalically oriented forces increase the cephalocaudal dimensions of the chest wall thus assisting inspiration. The effectiveness of these actions is reduced by physiologic (hyperinflation with increased lung volumes) and pathologic (emphysematous lungs) conditions.[18–20]

The diaphragmatic muscles are controlled by voluntary and autonomic neural pathways via the phrenic nerves and can respond to neural drive and workload. It has been shown that the diaphragm contracts against elastic resistive forces and returns to a constant resting position with each relaxation, with balance between the lung and chest wall recoil forces. Thus, expiration is partly effected by the elastic recoil of the thoracic walls and partly by the action of the abdominal muscles that push back the displaced abdominal viscera.

Although the diaphragm is known to be resistant to fatigue, diaphragmatic fatigue (defined by the loss of contractility and decreased duration of diaphragmatic contraction) can occur and is associated with unsuccessful weaning from mechanical ventilation.[21,22] A recent study by Levine and colleagues[21] demonstrated that prolonged mechanical ventilation with diaphragmatic inactivity caused diffuse atrophy of diaphragmatic muscle fibers. The diaphragms of brain-dead donors before organ harvest, who underwent mechanical ventilation for more than 18 hours, demonstrated marked decrease in slow-twitch type I and fast-twitch type II fibers when compared with diaphragms of control subjects who underwent elective thoracic surgery. It is also established that COPD patients have increased proportion of type I, fatigue-resistant fibers and a decreased proportion of type II, fatiguing fibers.[22] This fiber-type shift is thought to be a beneficial adaptive response to increased diaphragmatic loading.[23] The shift increases fatigue resistance but decreases force-generating capacity.[24] In summary, whereas several adaptation mechanisms might allow the diaphragm to continue to function adequately, inactivity of the diaphragm (as seen in ventilated patients or in various clinical conditions of diaphragmatic dysfunction or paralysis) can be rapidly associated with marked muscle atrophy and increased proteolysis.

The Role of the Diaphragm in Gastroesophageal Function

A detailed description of the gastroesophageal junction anatomy and mechanism is beyond the scope of this article (**Box 3**); a short description of the relationship between the diaphragmatic physiology and the functioning of the gastroesophageal area is warranted. Although the crural part of the diaphragm has a relatively smaller role in respiratory function when compared with the costal part, it plays an important part in gastroesophageal functions, including swallowing, vomiting, and preventing gastroesophageal reflux. The crural part relaxes for easy passage of a food bolus from the esophagus to the stomach in coordination with the esophageal peristalsis. The crural diaphragm temporarily ceases to contract when the esophagus distends with a food bolus, thus allowing food transition across the diaphragm.[25]

It is well recognized that the crural part plays an important role in emesis, which requires a complex orchestration of the abdominal muscles, gastrointestinal tract, respiratory muscles, and diaphragm.[4] In the retching phase of vomiting, costal and crural parts of the diaphragm contract

---

Box 3
The diaphragm in gastroesophageal function

- The crural part of the diaphragm is a major contributor for gastroesophageal functions.

- The relaxation of the crural diaphragm along with the extension of the esophagus with food bolus is necessary for smooth swallowing.

- Emesis requires a complex orchestration of the abdominal muscles, gastrointestional tract, respiratory muscles, and diaphragm.

- The crural diaphragm acts as an external sphincter of the esophagus to prevent acid reflux from the stomach.

---

strongly along with the abdominal muscles to increase the abdominal pressure while the gastroesophageal junction is tightly closed because of the contraction of the crural part of the diaphragm. During emesis (the expulsive phase), dissociation of the costal and crural muscles occurs. The costal diaphragm keeps contracting to produce increased abdominal pressure, whereas the crural diaphragm relaxes to allow the gastric contents to be ejected upwards. The coordination between the increased intra-abdominal pressure caused by rapid diaphragmatic descent, costal diaphragmatic contraction, and relaxation of the esophageal sphincters enables expulsive vomitting.[4]

The diaphragm functions as an antireflux barrier; the crural diaphragm serves as an external sphincter whereas the smooth muscle of the esophagus acts as an internal sphincter.[26] The crural diaphragm, an external sphincter producing an esophagogastric junction pressure, seems to grip the esophagus consistently and prevents acid reflux from the stomach.[3]

ACKNOWLEDGMENTS

We are indebted to Dennis Wei for his examplary artwork, to Roger Harris for his assistance in designing the figures, and to Basil Jardine for the radiologic images.

REFERENCES

1. Arora NS, Rochester DF. Effect of body weight and muscularity on human diaphragm muscle mass, thickness, and area. J Appl Phys 1982;52(1):64–70.
2. Pacia EB, Aldrich TK. Assessment of diaphragm function. Chest Surg Clin N Am 1998;8(2):225–36.
3. Schumpelick V, Steinau G, Schluper I, et al. Surgical embryology and anatomy of the diaphragm with surgical applications. Surg Clin North Am 2000; 80(1):213–39.

4. Pickering M, Jones JF. The diaphragm: two physiological muscles in one. J Anat 2002;201(4):305–12.

5. De Troyer A, Sampson M, Sigrist S, et al. The diaphragm: two muscles. Science 1981;213(4504):237–8.

6. Skandalakis PN, Skandalakis JE, Skandalakis LJ, et al. Surgical anatomy of the diaphragm. In: Fischer JE, Bland KI, editors. Mastery of surgery. 5th edition. Philadelphia: Lippincott Williams & Wilkins; 2006. p. 598–618.

7. Hussain SN, Magder S. Diaphragmatic intramuscular pressure in relation to tension, shortening, and blood flow. J Appl Phys 1991;71(1):159–67.

8. Robertson CH, Eschenbacher WL, Johnson RL, et al. Respiratory muscle blood flow distribution during expiratory resistance. J Clin Invest 1977;60: 473–80.

9. Supinski GS, DiMarco AF, Altose MD. Effect of diaphragmatic contraction on intramuscular pressure and vascular impedance. J Appl Phys 1990;68(4): 1486–93.

10. Buchler B, Magder S, Katsardis H, et al. Effects of pleural pressure and abdominal pressure on diaphragmatic blood flow. J Appl Phys 1985;58(3):691–7.

11. Venuta F, Rendina EA. Diaphragm: anatomy, embryology, pathophysiology. In: Patterson GA, Pearson FG, Cooper JD, et al, editors. Pearson's thoracic and esophageal surgery. 3rd edition. St. Louis (MO): Elsevier; 2008. p. 1367–79.

12. Fell SC. Surgical anatomy of the diaphragm and the phrenic nerve. Chest Surg Clin N Am 1998;8(2): 281–94.

13. Kirchner PA. Porous diaphragmatic syndromes. Chest Surg Clin N Am 1998;8:449–72.

14. De Troyer A, Estenne M. Functional anatomy of the respiratory muscles. Clin Chest Med 1988;9(2): 175–93.

15. Rochester DF. The diaphragm: contractile properties and fatigue. J Clin Invest 1985;75(5):1397–402.

16. Lieberman DA, Faulkner JA, Craig AB Jr, et al. Performance and histochemical composition of guinea pig and human diaphragm. J Appl Phys 1973;34(2):233–7.

17. Geiger PC, Cody MJ, Macken RL, et al. Maximum specific force depends on myosin heavy chain content in rat diaphragm muscle fibers. J Appl Phys 2000;89(2):695–703.

18. Poole DC, Sexton WL, Farkas GA, et al. Diaphragm structure and function in health and disease. Med Sci Sports Exerc 1997;29(6):738–54.

19. Brochard L, Harf A, Lorino H, et al. Inspiratory pressure support prevents diaphragmatic fatigue during weaning from mechanical ventilation. Am Rev Respir Dis 1989;139(2):513–21.

20. Pourriat JL, Lamberto C, Hoang PH, et al. Diaphragmatic fatigue and breathing pattern during weaning from mechanical ventilation in COPD patients. Chest 1986;90(5):703–7.

21. Levine S, Nguyen T, Taylor N, et al. Rapid disuse atrophy of diaphragm fibers in mechanically ventilated humans. N Engl J Med 2008;358(13): 1327–35.

22. Barreiro E, de la Puente B, Minguella J, et al. Oxidative stress and respiratory muscle dysfunction in severe chronic obstructive pulmonary disease. Am J Respir Crit Care Med 2005; 171(10):1116–24.

23. Ottenheijm CA, Heunks LM, Dekhuijzen PN. Diaphragm muscle fiber dysfunction in chronic obstructive pulmonary disease: toward a pathophysiological concept. Am J Respir Crit Care Med 2007; 175(12):1233–40.

24. Levine S, Nguyen T, Kaiser LR, et al. Human diaphragm remodeling associated with chronic obstructive pulmonary disease: clinical implications. Am J Respir Crit Care Med 2003;168(6):706–13.

25. Miller AD. Respiratory muscle control during vomiting. Can J Physiol Pharmacol 1990;68(2):237–41.

26. Mittal RK. The crural diaphragm, an external lower esophageal sphincter: a definitive study. Gastroenterology 1993;105(5):1565–7.

Imaging the Diaphragm

Heidi C. Roberts, MD

KEYWORDS

• Diaphragm • Motion • Paralysis • Hernia • Eventration

The diaphragm is a thin, fibromuscular structure providing two entirely different yet equally important functions in the human body: it serves as a mechanical barrier between the pleural and abdominal cavities and maintains the pressure gradient between those two cavities, and even more importantly, the diaphragm performs most of the respiratory work.

Given its location between the chest and abdominal cavities, it is depicted on thoracic and abdominal scans. However, because of its complex structure and complex function, and because of its thinness and mostly tangential course that evades delineation on axial, cross-sectional imaging, it is not typically visualized in its entirety and no comments are made on it routinely.

Most diaphragmatic processes are asymptomatic, and it is not uncommon that an abnormality of the diaphragmatic position, contour, or structure is incidentally seen on thoracic or abdominal scans performed for a different reason.

This issue describes the normal and abnormal position, motion, and morphology of the diaphragm, on chest radiography and fluoroscopy, but also on computed tomography (CT), magnetic resonance imaging (MRI), and ultrasound.

IMAGING TECHNIQUES

There are both static and dynamic imaging techniques performed to image the hemidiaphragms, and the appearance of the different diaphragmatic conditions will be described in the according sections.

Chest radiographs serve most commonly as the starting point, both for expected as well as unexpected diaphragmatic conditions (**Table 1**). The position of the diaphragm is indirectly interpreted from the inferior level of the lungs. If an abnormality is seen, or suspected, further imaging may be chosen to either better display the structure and morphology of the diaphragm, or to yield functional information on the diaphragmatic motion during the respiratory cycle. Limited information may be available from a chest radiograph in inspiration and expiration.

Both computed tomography (CT) and magnetic resonance imaging (MRI) may be used to display the diaphragmatic morphology. Coronal reconstructions of CT scans or coronal images of MRI scans allow a similar assessment of the diaphragmatic position as chest radiography does, and in addition yield direct delineation of the diaphragmatic muscle. MRI has the added advantage that dynamic scanning allows assessment of the diaphragmatic motion,[1] but this does not offset the inherent disadvantages of MRI (accessibility, time, and costs) that make it a second-line tool used to study the diaphragm.[2]

Dynamic imaging evaluating the diaphragmatic motion can be performed with ultrasound or fluoroscopy. Both technologies allow a visualization of the motion during the normal respiratory cycle, or during forced inspiration. Fluoroscopy in frontal projection is limited by the small field of view, which is only large enough to either display one diaphragm or the medial portions only of both diaphragms, and oblique or lateral positioning may be better to assess both diaphragms simultaneously.[2] Ultrasound is a valuable alternative to fluoroscopy providing a similar assessment of the diaphragmatic motion.[3–5] Its advantages include portability, as well as a simultaneous assessment of the diaphragmatic structure and thickness.[4,5] The main disadvantages of ultrasound are the small field of view, and in particular the left diaphragm maybe difficult to visualize in the presence of obesity or gaseous distension, and ultrasound is chosen only when fluoroscopy

Department of Medical Imaging, University Health Network/Mt. Sinai Hospital/Women's College Hospital, 76 Grenville Street, Room W2 72, Toronto, ON M5S 1B2, Canada
E-mail address: heidi.roberts@uhn.on.ca

Thorac Surg Clin 19 (2009) 431–450
doi:10.1016/j.thorsurg.2009.08.008
1547-4127/09/$ – see front matter © 2009 Elsevier Inc. All rights reserved.

thoracic.theclinics.com

Table 1
Using chest radiographs as the most common starting point for diaphragmatic abnormalities, typical findings and their possible diagnosis are listed, as well as the further procedures to obtain diagnostic confirmation

Position and Contour of the Diaphragm	Possible Diagnosis	Diagnostic Confirmation
High, unilateral	Elevation, 2nd to lung disease elevation, 2nd to abdominal disease paralysis	History, CT of the lungs, PFTs history, abdominal u/s sniff test (paradixocal movement), CT (phrenic nerve involvement) history (eg, recent cardiac surgery)
High, bilateral	Elevation, 2nd to lung disease elevation, 2nd to obesity weakness	History, CT of the lungs, PFTs history, physical examination history (prolonged ventilation)
Flat	2nd to lung disease (COPD)	History, PFTs
Focal bulge	Eventration hernia traumatic hernia neoplasm	Typical location, history (no symptoms) typical location (hiatus, foramen of Bochdalek or Morgagni), CT history (acute or remote trauma), serial chest radiographs, CT/MRI CT/MRI

Abbreviations: COPD, chronic obstructive pulmonary disease; PFT, pulmonary function test.

cannot be performed or cannot be interpreted owing to diaphragm obscuration from adjacent pleural fluid or parenchymal consolidation.[2] Diaphragmatic motion abnormalities might become evident only during forced inspiration, which is assessed during the so-called sniff test. During the "sniffing," the patient inhales rapidly and sharply through the nose with the mouth closed, and the diaphragmatic motion is observed with either fluoroscopy or ultrasound.

Diaphragmatic Position

The position of the hemidiaphragms is easily and efficiently assessed on chest radiographs. The normal diaphragm forms a smooth dome, its superior aspect outlined by the adjacent air-containing lung, with the exception of the medial portion of the left hemidiaphragm, which may be obscured by the adjacent heart. The inferior surface of the diaphragm is not visible, as it is obscured by the adjacent liver on the right and gastric wall on the left, and the diaphragmatic position on chest radiographs is inferred from the inferior level of the lungs.

Normal Diaphragmatic Position

On postero-anterior (PA) chest radiographs, the level of the dome of the right diaphragms projects over the anterior 5th or 6th rib,[6,7] and the posterior 10th rib.[7] In almost all healthy individuals, the left diaphragm has a lower position than the right and its dome projects up to one rib interspace below the right one (**Fig. 1A**).[6–9] In up to 10% of

healthy subjects, both diaphragmatic domes are at the same height, and might be difficult to be differentiated on the lateral view, hence other signs are needed to identify the diaphragms on the lateral view: the anterior left diaphragm is obscured by the adjacent heart, there might be air under the left diaphragm in the stomach or splenic colon flexure, and the major fissure arising from the left diaphragm is typically steeper than the right.

Eventration

On chest radiographs, both a partial and a total eventration can be identified.

A partial eventration is a common incidental finding in individuals 60 years or older, typically occurring in the anteromedial portion of the right diaphragm (**Fig. 1B**). As it is of no clinical significance, no further imaging needs to be initiated.[8,10] In rare instances, a partial eventration needs to be differentiated from a tumor or hernia, and CT or MRI may be used to determine the nature of the bulge.[11] The underlying diaphragmatic anomaly is congenital; it is an incomplete muscular development of all or part of one or both hemidiaphragms.[12] During aging, the continual displacement of the diaphragm by negative intrathoracic and positive intra-abdominal pressures results in a progressive stretching and weakening of the affected portions, eventually causing it to bulge.[13,14]

Total eventration of the diaphragm is indistinguishable from a diaphragmatic paralysis (see

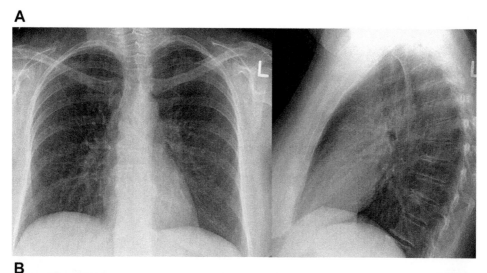

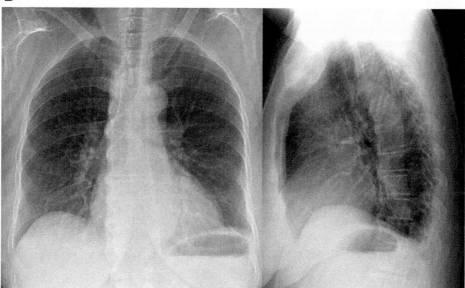

Fig. 1. (*A*) PA and lateral chest radiograph of normal hemidiaphragms. The dome of the right diaphragm is at the level of the 5th anterior and 10th posterior rib, the dome of the left diaphragm is about one inter-rib space deeper. (*B*) PA and lateral chest radiograph of a partial eventration of the right anterior diaphragm. The anteromedial right diaphragm demonstrates a broad, smooth upward bulging. (*C*) PA and lateral chest radiograph of unilateral elevation of the left diaphragm. Note that there is no atelectasis of the adjacent lung (as opposed to paralysis, see **Fig. 2**). (*D*) PA and lateral chest radiograph of inverted diaphragms as a result of severe COPD.

later in this article) on chest radiographs. As a differentiating sign, a diaphragmatic eventration will typically not have adjacent areas of atelectatic lung, whereas paralysis of the diaphragm will. This is because the eventrated diaphragm still moves downward with inspiration, but a paralyzed diaphragm does not. Total eventration is rare in adults, occurs mostly on the left side, and is associated with severe respiratory symptoms and respiratory failure.[12,15] During fluoroscopy, an eventrated diaphragm typically displays an

inspiratory lag followed by delayed downward motion,[12] but there may be slight paradoxic, little, or no movement, and in these cases it may be indistinguishable from diaphragmatic paralysis even during dynamic imaging.[9,12]

Elevation

On chest radiographs, a diaphragmatic elevation appears identical to a diaphragmatic paralysis. The underling abnormality however lies outside

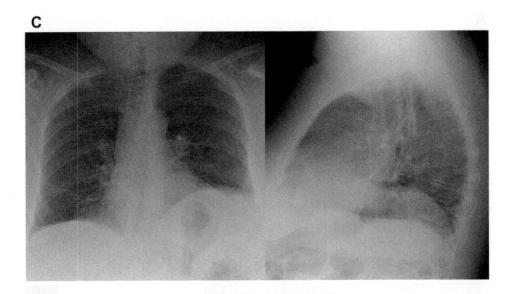

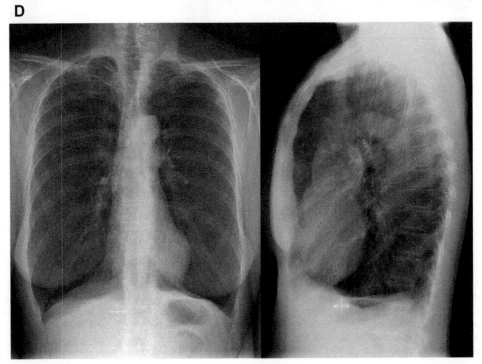

Fig. 1. (*continued*)

of the diaphragm and is usually found in the lungs: the diaphragms are passively elevated following insufficient inspiratory effort because of obesity,[16] or decreased lung volumes resulting from diffuse interstitial fibrosis, atelectasis, surgical resection, or tumors such as malignant pleural mesothelioma.[17–19] As a lung disease can affect one or both lungs, diaphragmatic elevation can be unilateral or bilateral (**Fig. 1**C). Unilateral elevation of the diaphragm may also passively result from abdominal disease such as hepatomegaly, masses, fluid collections, or bowel distension. Other causes of uni- or bilateral diaphragmatic elevation are pain as a result of rib fractures, pleurisy, pneumonia, or acute abdominal inflammations such as cholecystitis. As the diaphragmatic motion is not affected, adjacent atelectasis of the lung is uncommon, as opposed to diaphragmatic paralysis. The normal motion during the respiratory cycle and forced inspiration can be assessed with fluoroscopy and confirm the diagnosis of passive diaphragmatic elevation.

Flattening

In this condition the diaphragm loses its dome shape and appears flattened or even inverted on chest radiographs (**Fig. 1**D). Just as in diaphragmatic elevation, this is a passive process in this case owing to increased lung volumes, most commonly as a result of emphysema, but less commonly because of tension pneumothorax, or other lung diseases such as cystic fibrosis, histiocytosis X, or lymphangioleiomyomatosis.[2] As these parenchymal diseases are typically bilateral, diaphragmatic flattening most frequently involves both hemidiaphragms.

DIAPHRAGMATIC MOTION
Normal Diaphragmatic Motion

As mentioned previously, the diaphragmatic position is easily assessed on chest radiographs, but an abnormal position results from passive elevation or depression of the diaphragms as well as from genuine conditions of the diaphragmatic motion. Normally, both diaphragms descend symmetrically during inspiration and ascend symmetrically during expiration, a movement that is accentuated during the sniff test.[2] The range of diaphragmatic motion is highly variable among healthy subjects, depends on the individual training and abdominal muscle recruitment, but does not relate to the vital capacity of the lungs. In healthy individuals, the excursion of the domes of the diaphragm averages 3 to 5 cm but ranges from 2 to 10 cm.[20–24] Normal diaphragmatic motion however has a considerable overlap with abnormal motion and makes interpretation of dynamic diaphragmatic assessment difficult, as unequal excursion is common (typically differs less than 1.5 cm and does not have a side preference[6,8,21]), minimal paradoxic inspiratory motion may be observed, and the dome of the diaphragm may move differently from the rest of the diaphragm.[25] False positives and false negative findings are seen during forced inspiration, ie, during the sniff test[15,20]; also paradoxic motion during the sniff test is common. As such, an abnormal interpretation of the diaphragmatic motion requires a paradoxic movement of at least 2 cm.[26]

Diaphragmatic Weakness and Fatigue

On chest radiographs, a weak diaphragm appears abnormally high. On fluoroscopy, particularly during the sniff test, there is a normal direction

but decreased amplitude of diaphragmatic excursion. Diaphragmatic weakness describes the lack of muscular strength to perform adequate ventilation, which often is a reversible consequence from prolonged ventilatory support. Diaphragmatic fatigue describes the inability to maintain the work required for adequate ventilation,[27] for example resulting from increased respiratory effort in chronic lung disease.

Diaphragmatic Paralysis

On chest radiographs, a paralyzed diaphragm displays an accentuated dome configuration, with deepened and narrowed costophrenic and costovertebral sulci.[11] In the case of a paralyzed left hemidiaphragm, the stomach and the splenic flexure typically contain more gas than normal (**Fig. 2**).[11] In contrast to diaphragmatic elevation, adjacent atelectasis is common. However, these signs are unreliable, and both unilateral and bilateral diaphragmatic paralysis is usually indistinguishable from the previously mentioned abnormalities of the diaphragmatic position or motion. Further imaging traditionally involves assessment of the diaphragmatic motion, which is more reliable in unilateral than in bilateral paralysis. In unilateral paralysis, the paralyzed hemidiaphragm follows passively the pressure changes in the pleural and abdominal spaces, thus paradoxically moving upward during inspiration and downward during expiration.[12,23] The sniff test is positive in more than 90% of patients with unilateral phrenic

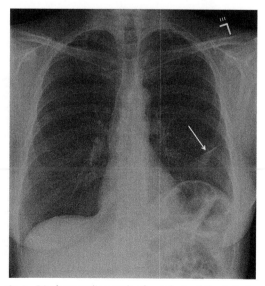

Fig. 2. PA chest radiograph of paralysis of the left diaphragm. The stomach and the splenic colon flexure contain more gas than normal, and there is atelectasis in the adjacent parenchyma (*arrow*).

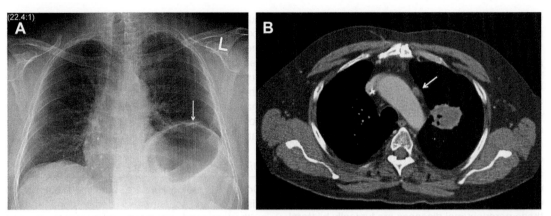

Fig. 3. PA chest radiograph (*A*) shows an elevated left diaphragm, the adjacent atelectasis suggests a phrenic paralysis (*arrow*). (*B*) Axial CT scan of bronchogenic carcinoma in the left upper lobe and a lymph node metastasis (*arrow*) in the presumed location of the phrenic nerve, likely responsible for the paralysis.

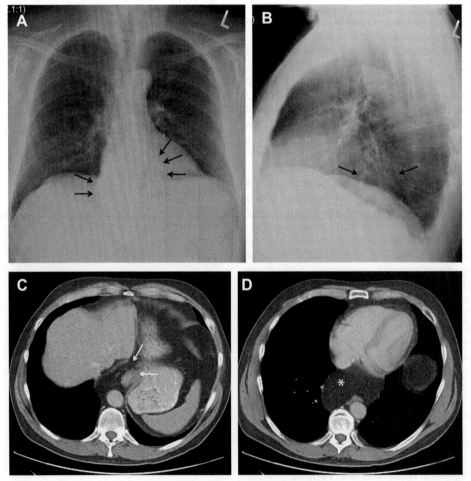

Fig. 4. PA (*A*) and lateral chest (*B*) radiograph of a hiatus hernia. It displays as a soft tissue mass seen in the retro-cardiac space (*arrows*). Even without an air-fluid-level indicating the position of the stomach, this appearance is typical for a hiatus hernia. The CT scan at the level of the esophageal hiatus shows the wide opening of the hiatus (*arrows* in *C*), and sliding of the stomach into the thorax. Most of the hernia contains fat (*asterisk* in *D*).

nerve palsy.[15,28] Fluoroscopic tests of bilateral diaphragmatic paralysis are difficult and sometimes misleading:[25] dynamic imaging displays paradoxic upward motion of both hemidiaphragms during the sniff test with inward rather than normal outward movement of the abdominal wall,[25,29] but as the paradoxic movement relies on the action of a functioning contralateral hemidiaphragm, this may be difficult to detect. False negative sniff tests might be found when accessory muscles result in a cranial movement of the ribs and an apparent decrease in the diaphragmatic position during forced inspiration.[20,30]

The interpretation of dynamic imaging in suspected diaphragmatic paralysis is limited, showing overlap between complete eventration and paralysis,[17] overlap between weakness and paralysis,[12] and overlap with limited motion in severe chronic obstructive pulmonary disease (COPD),[2] or weak or debilitated patients,[2] as we rely on their compliance and cooperation. Moreover, only indirect information can be expected from the assessment of the diaphragmatic motion. As the underlying reason for the diaphragmatic paralysis is typically a pathologic process involving the phrenic nerve, a tool directly assessing the presence or nature of an abnormality along the course of the nerve is advantageous. Consequently, dynamic imaging has almost entirely been replaced by CT for the assessment of a diaphragmatic paralysis

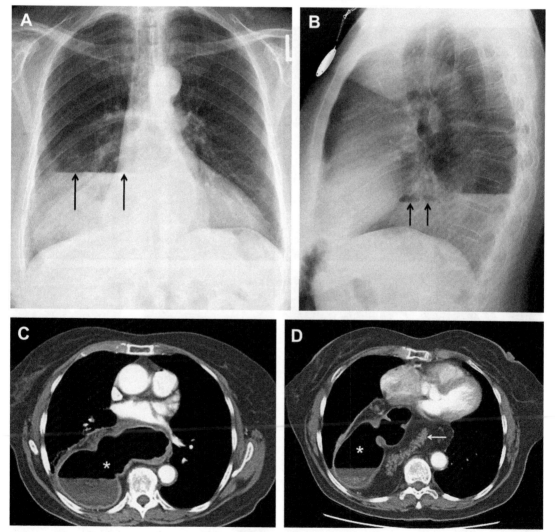

Fig. 5. PA (*A*) and lateral chest (*B*) radiograph and axial CT scans (*C, D*) of a large hiatus hernia. The chest radiographs show a large mass in the right posterior hemithorax with one large (*arrows* in *A*) and several small (*arrows* in *B*) air fluid levels. The CT scans reveal the extent of the herniation, containing fat, omentum, stomach (*asterisk* in *C* and *D*), and pancreas (*arrow* in *D*).

suspected on chest radiographs. An evaluation of the cause of a diaphragmatic paralysis may lie anywhere from the brainstem to the diaphragm itself; however, the most common cause of a phrenic nerve irritation is bronchogenic carcinoma or other malignancy, which accounts for approximately one third of cases, and can be easily detected on CT scans (**Fig. 3**). CT is performed to exclude a treatable cause such as a tumor or an aneurysm, and to differentiate it from a spontaneously reversible cause such as a hypothermic injury of the phrenic nerve following cardiac surgery[15] or a postinfectious state, poliomyelitis, and so forth.[2,15]

Other, more rare, abnormalities of the diaphragmatic motion include involuntary and irregular contractions that can be diagnosed on fluoroscopy. Flutter has been described as contractions occurring with a rate of 35 to 480 times per minute, on average 150,[31–33] whereas hiccups occur in a lower frequency than flutter, at a rate of 6 to 100 times per minute.[31–33] On fluoroscopy, all or parts of one or both hemidiaphragms may be affected.

DIAPHRAGMATIC HERNIATION

Diaphragmatic herniations, or hernias, describe the intrathoracic protrusion of intra-abdominal or retroperitoneal tissue and organs via diaphragmatic defects. Diaphragmatic hernias are commonly seen first on chest radiographs, frequently as an incidental finding. They present as an abnormal contour bulging the diaphragm and, if large, may

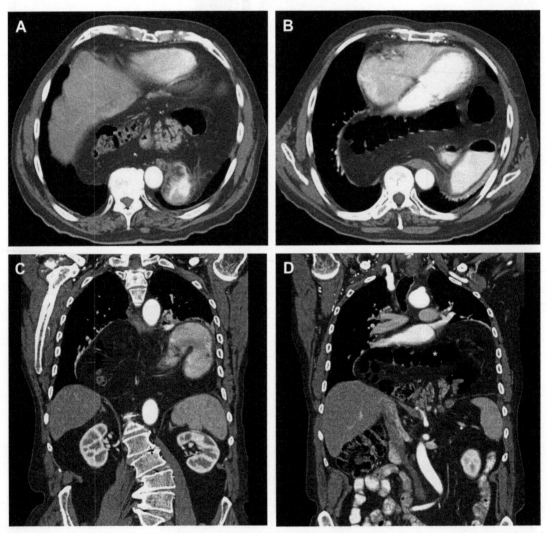

Fig. 6. Axial CT scans (*A, B*) and coronal reconstructions (*C, D*) of a large hiatus hernia containing stomach and large bowel (*asterisk* in *D*). The location of the different organs in the chest is easier appreciated on the reconstruction.

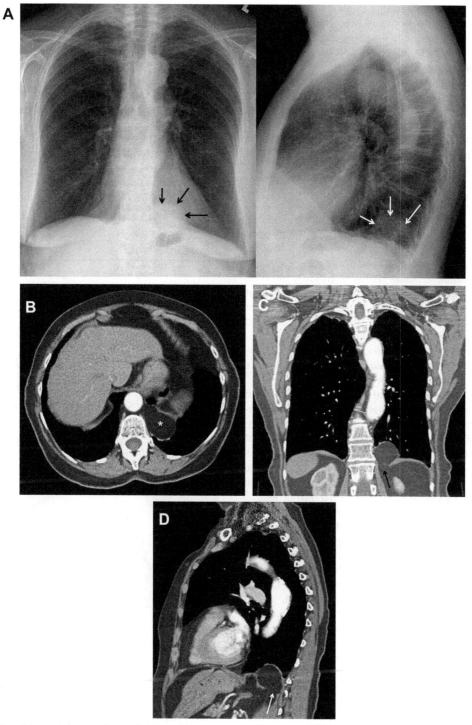

Fig. 7. PA and lateral chest radiograph (*A*) and CT scan of a Bochdalek hernia. The chest radiograph shows a well-defined soft tissue mass bulging from the posterior aspect of the left hemidiaphragm (*arrows*). The axial CT scan (*B*) demonstrates the fatty content of this "mass" (*asterisk*). The coronal and sagittal reconstructions (*C, D*) best display the diaphragmatic defect (*arrows*).

be indistinguishable from an elevated diaphragm. The documentation of the presence, extent, and content of a hernia is equally possible with either CT or MRI, but CT with coronal and sagittal reformations is the most efficient diagnostic tool for the evaluation of diaphragmatic hernias.[34]

Diaphragmatic defects may occur in natural foramina or congenitally weak areas, and result in hernias that can be seen in typical locations, or may result from previous trauma and as such can be seen anywhere along the diaphragmatic contour.

Esophageal/Hiatus Hernia

Hiatus hernias are common incidental findings on chest radiographs, in particular in the elderly population; the incidence increases with age to 65% between the ages of 60 and 79 years.[35] On chest radiographs, a hiatus hernia is typically seen as a retrocardiac soft tissue mass, with or without an air-fluid level (**Fig. 4**). In the case of a larger defect, when most of the stomach has herniated into the chest, the stomach may undergo a volvolus, resulting in the presence of a larger mass containing a double air-fluid level. Incarceration as well as strangulation may occur.[36]

On CT, the esophageal hiatus can be delineated as on opening just to the left of the midline, marginated by the right and left diaphragmatic crura. Occasionally, the splitting of the medial fibers of the right crus and the left crus can be seen as well. The esophageal hiatus has an elliptical shape, and the distance between the medial margins of the crura should be 15 mm or less.[11] This hiatus is a congenitally weak area, which can widen in the presence of increased intra-abdominal pressure or obesity. Sliding hernias (see **Fig. 4**) are much more common than para-esophageal hernias, in which the stomach herniates up alongside the lower esophagus.[2] CT will demonstrate the contents of the hernia, which may contain fat (see **Fig 4**) or the stomach alone, or, if the defect is large, other organs such as the transverse colon, omentum, liver, or pancreas (**Figs. 5** and **6**).[37] Multiplanar reconstructions are helpful to assess the entry into the chest, in particular for presurgical planning (see **Fig. 6**).

Bochdalek Hernia

On chest radiographs, a Bochdalek hernia manifests as an asymptomatic posterior mediastinal mass in the typical posteromedial aspect of either hemidiaphragm. A Bochdalek hernia occurs through a congenitally weak area, the pleuroperitoneal canal, and becomes manifest during aging, in the presence of obesity and emphysema. The

prevalence has been reported as up to 35% in individuals 70 years or older.[35,38] Owing to the protective effect of the liver, Bochdalek hernias are more common on the left than right.[17,39] Although the radiographic appearance is suggestive of a Bochdalek hernia, it may be indistinguishable from a pulmonary or paravertebral mass. Diagnostic confirmation and documentation of hernia content is easily possible with CT (**Fig. 7**).[40,41] The defect can be seen in typical location in the posterior diaphragmatic region lateral to the crura. In the adult population, most Bochdalek hernias contain perinephric fat. If they are large, they may contain kidney, or rarely stomach and small bowel.[12,42]

Morgagni Hernia

On chest radiographs, a Morgagni hernia usually manifests as a smooth, well-defined opacity in the right more often then in the left cardiophrenic angle (the left side is protected by the heart), typically displaying a homogeneous density. An inhomogeneous density indicates an air-containing loop of bowel in the hernia.[43] Morgagni hernias are uncommon, and may be seen as incidental findings detected on chest radiographs. Similar to the hiatus or Bochdalek hernias, the underlying

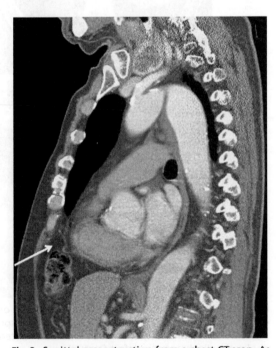

Fig. 8. Sagittal reconstruction from a chest CT scan. As an incidental finding, a small amount of fat is seen protruding into the right cardiophrenic angle, the weakness of the sternal portion of the diaphragm can be appreciated as well (*arrow*).

defect is congenital and results from a developmental failure of the fibrotendinous elements of the sternal part of the diaphragm to fuse with the costal part, which manifests itself as a defect in the presence of increased abdominal pressure or obesity. Morgagni hernias can be seen in various sizes (**Fig. 8**). The radiographic appearance may resemble any other cardiophrenic angle mass, including a pericardial cyst, pericardial fat pads, lymphadenopathy, or other masses (**Fig. 9**). On CT, the diagnosis and extent of a Morgagni hernia can be easily documented by the presence of fat (see **Fig. 9**) or abdominal contents between the costal and sternal attachments of the diaphragm

A

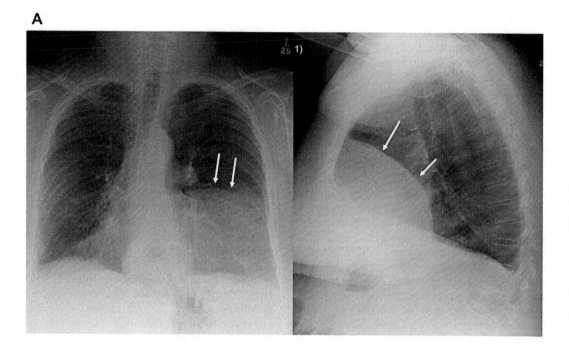

B

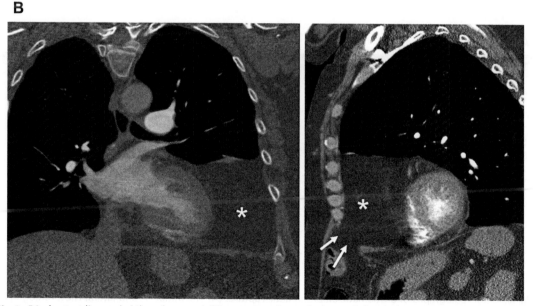

Fig. 9. PA chest radiograph (*A*) and coronal CT reconstructions of a large, left-sided Morgagni hernia. The chest radiographs show a large mass, in left paracardial location (*arrows*), with obscuration of the heart border. The CT scans demonstrate that this "mass" contains entirely of fat (*asterisk*) and also reveal the diaphragmatic defect (*arrows*). (*Images courtesy of* Dr Elsie Nguyen.)

in the right anteromedial location, and the hernia may contain omentum or transverse colon, stomach, liver, or small bowel.[11,12,44,45]

Traumatic Diaphragmatic Hernia

Traumatic diaphragmatic hernias represent a diagnostic challenge not only clinically but also radiographically. They do not have a typical location, as the underlying trauma might have affected any portion of the diaphragms. They may occur acutely but also years after the trauma and the remote history might not be known at the time the chest radiograph is read.

The chest radiographic findings of an acute diaphragmatic rupture are nonspecific and may include an unusual air-fluid level in the lower chest, and abnormally irregular diaphragmatic contour, an unexplained contralateral mediastinal shift, or an unexplained high position of the stomach that may be seen directly or indirectly by the location of a nasogastric tube above the level of the diaphragm (**Fig. 10**).[46–50] Penetrating injuries do not have a side preference, but ruptures as a result of blunt trauma occur mostly on the left.[51,52] A chronic rupture may be asymptomatic or produce only mild, nonspecific symptoms for years, such as vague abdominal distress, chest or shoulder pain, or recurrent pneumonia. Over time, the resulting weakened area at the site of rupture increases with the constant transdiaphragmatic pressure gradient, eventually resulting in

a herniation.[53] Only about one third of ruptures are diagnosed promptly, most have a delayed presentation. Comparison with serial previous chest radiographs may show a growing diaphragmatic mass that could be confused with an eventration, a hiatus hernia, a tumor, abscess, or cyst. In general, chest radiographs have a low sensitivity in the diagnosis of a traumatic diaphragmatic hernia, lowest in right-sided rupture or perforating injury.[46–48] The knowledge of the patient's recent or remote trauma history is crucial for correct interpretation of the radiographic findings. Diaphragmatic rupture has been reported in only 0.5% to 6.0% of blunt trauma survivors,[54–58] but the patient ought to be able to remember the event, as a diaphragmatic rupture from a blunt trauma usually requires a considerable and sudden increase in the pleuroperitoneal pressure gradient, typically from a fall, an automobile accident, and only rarely from an event that is too minor to be recalled by the patient.[59,60] Most diaphragmatic ruptures result from a blunt trauma (75%), less from a penetrating injury (25%).[46]

As these findings are nonspecific, the trauma history in combination with unexplained radiographic findings should lead to a prompt CT or MRI, which can confirm the diaphragmatic rupture and lead to timely surgical correction.[52,61] The sharp discontinuity of the diaphragm might be directly visualized, as well as the intrathoracic organ positioning. Traumatic herniations may present with various sizes, and a hernia resulting

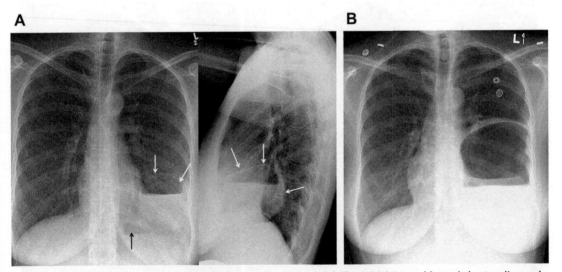

Fig. 10. Chest radiographs of a traumatic diaphragmatic rupture. (*A*) The initial PA and lateral chest radiographs show a large mass with an air-fluid level (*white arrows*), which on the lateral view resembles a hiatus hernia, but on the PA view is separate from the esophageal hiatus (*black arrow*). The mass obscures the diaphragm. A follow-up portable chest radiograph a few hours later shows marked increase in the air-filled mass, with mediastinal shift (*B*).

from a blunt trauma is usually larger than a hernia resulting from a penetrating trauma.[62] Herniations most commonly involve the stomach on the left, and the liver on the right, but can also include the large or small bowel, omentum, liver, or spleen.[55–57] CT has a high sensitivity in the detection of traumatic diaphragmatic ruptures, reported between 60% and 95%.[52,63–67] In diagnostically challenging cases the direct multiplanar imaging of MRI might be helpful.[68]

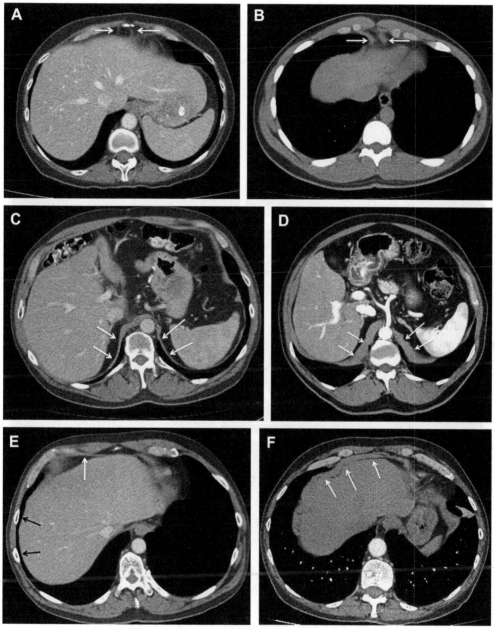

Fig. 11. Normal appearance of the hemidiaphragms on CT (different patients). Thin (*A*) or thick (*B*) appearance of the sternal portions, arising from the xyphoid (*arrows*). Thin (*C*) or thick (*D*) appearance of diaphragmatic crura (*arrows*). The typically smooth costal diaphragm is inseparable from the adjacent organs in the absence of separating fat (*black arrows* in *E*), but can be delineated when a fat layer is present (*white arrows* in *E, F*). On contrast-enhanced CT scans, a smooth costal diaphragm remains low in density and thus can be separated from the enhancing liver (*arrows* in *G*). Nodular (*H*) and linear (*I*) indentation of the diaphragm from the costal portion of the diaphragm (*arrows*). Owing to its thinness and isodensity to the liver and spleen, the normal diaphragmatic domes are not separable from the adjacent organs—liver, spleen or stomach, on coronal (*J*) or sagittal (*K*) reconstructions (*arrows*).

DIAPHRAGMATIC STRUCTURE
Normal Diaphragmatic Structure

The normal diaphragm cannot be delineated on chest radiographs, but is equally well appreciated on CT or MRI, as well we on ultrasound.

On CT scans, the diaphragms have soft tissue density, which separates them from the low-density air above and the low-density fat below. As the diaphragms are thin and isodense to the soft tissue organs of the upper abdomen, ie, the liver, spleen, stomach, or colon, they are not

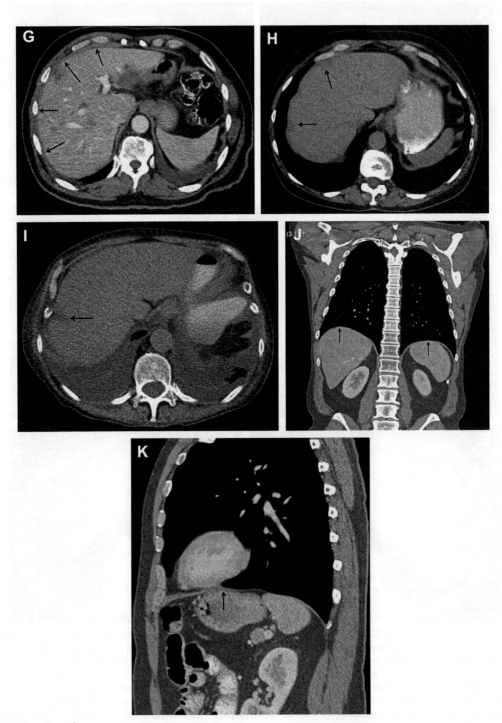

Fig. 11. (continued)

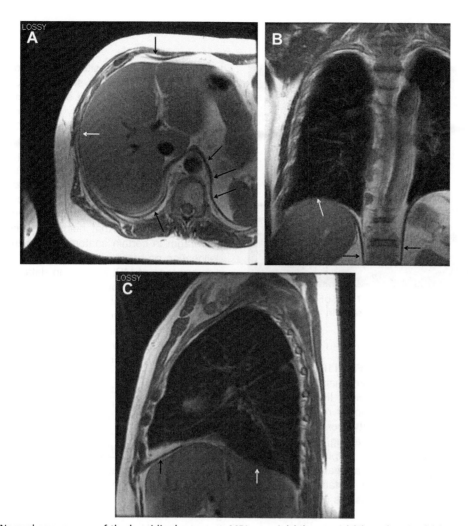

Fig. 12. Normal appearance of the hemidiaphragms on MRI on axial (*A*), coronal (*B*), and sagittal (*C*) images. The muscular diaphragm is isointense to liver and spleen and thus inseparable from these organs (*white arrows*), but easily identified in the presence of fat (*black arrows*).

visible in areas where there is no adjacent fat, in particular along the diaphragmatic domes.[69,70]

The anterior, sternal portion arises from the back of the xyphoid, and may be of different thickness (**Fig. 11**A, B). If this area is nodular, it may be confused with precardial lymph nodes, the distinction however can be easily made during scrolling or on multiplanar reconstructions.[69]

Easily visualized are also the posterolateral regions of the diaphragms and the diaphragmatic crura, which are the most vertical parts of the diaphragms and thus most commonly visible on cross-sectional imaging. They also can vary considerably in thickness in healthy subjects, and may be smooth or nodular (**Fig. 11**C, D).[71–73]

The costal portion of the diaphragms arise from the lower six ribs and their cartilages is most difficult to appreciate on cross-sectional imaging. They are commonly smooth, aligned along and inseparable from the liver and spleen on noncontrast images (**Fig. 11**E), but can be identified

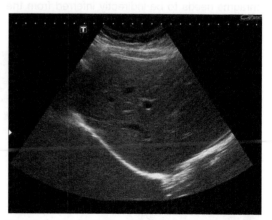

Fig. 13. Normal ultrasound appearance of the diaphragm: it has a similar echogenicity to the liver and chest wall muscles (*arrow*), and is separated from these structures by thin, echogenic lines. These lines represent the facial planes along the chest wall muscles, peritoneal surface and liver capsule, with fat within these tissue interfaces.

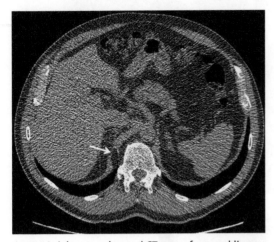

Fig. 14. Axial, non-enhanced CT scan of a crural lipoma shows a fat attenuation lesion in the right crus (*arrow*).

when a fat layer is present (**Fig. 11**F). On postcontrast scans, the diaphragm maintains a lower density than the enhancing liver or spleen (**Fig. 11**G),[74] or it may appear relatively hyperdense to a low-density, fatty liver. Depending on the degree of inspiration, training, age, and other individual differences, the diaphragm however might be more nodular in appearance, resulting in indentations of the liver surface that can be confused with focal liver lesions (**Fig. 11**H, I), on axial images, but can be easily resolved with scrolling or multiplanar reformations.[72]

Toward the dome, the diaphragm is imaged tangentially on cross-sectional scans, and more difficult to evaluate. The position of the diaphragms needs to be indirectly inferred from the

known characteristic positioning of the diaphragm between the surrounding structures. Coronal or sagittal reconstructions are only of limited help, as the thin diaphragm directly abuts the adjacent isodense soft tissue organs (**Fig. 11**J, K).

On MRI, the normal diaphragmatic structure displays low signal intensity on all sequences. It is of similar signal intensity to the liver and spleen and, as on CT, best seen when a fat layer separates the diaphragm from the adjacent organs (**Fig. 12**).[75] Advantages of MRI include the direct multiplanar imaging that helps to delineate the diaphragm in certain anatomic areas that evade delineation on cross-sectional images. The main disadvantage of MRI is the long data acquisition that typically does not allow breathold and results in motion artifacts obscuring a detailed assessment of the diaphragmatic structure.

Because of the initially mentioned limitations, mainly small field of view and difficult visualization in the presence of gas and in obese patients, ultrasound is hardly ever used to evaluate the diaphragmatic structure. The normal diaphragms display the typical intermediate echogenicity of skeletal muscle (**Fig. 13**).

Diaphragmatic Neoplasms

On chest radiographs, small diaphragmatic neoplasms are not visualized and large tumors demonstrate a focal bulge that may be indistinguishable from a diaphragmatic hernia, eventration, or pleural lesion.[1]

Primary neoplasms of the diaphragm are rare.[76–80] They are most commonly benign, and include lipomas (**Fig. 14**),[35,44,81] neural tumors, leiomyomas, hemangiomas, or other soft tissue

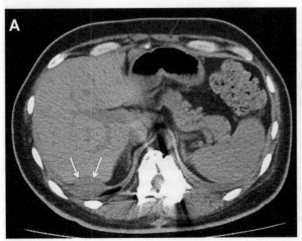
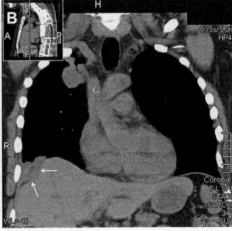

Fig. 15. Contrast-enhanced CT images of diaphragmatic metastases from a sarcoma show abnormal, focal thickening of the right hemidiaphragm (*arrows*).

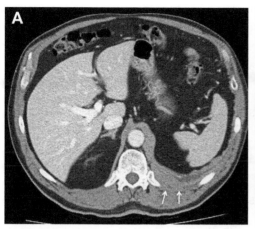
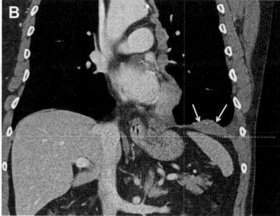

Fig. 16. Contrast-enhanced CT scan of a left-sided metastasizing mesothelioma. Soft tissue nodules are seen along the left diaphragm (*arrows*). On coronal reconstructions, the diaphragm is inseparable, suggesting infiltration of the diaphragm.

tumors. Lipomas may be seen incidentally and display their typical, low density of fat attenuation on CT.[44] Malignant primary neoplasms are even more uncommon, and include fibrosarcomas.[77] Non-neoplastic abnormalities have been reported as well and include lymphangiomas and endometriomata.

Secondary neoplasms of the diaphragms include lymphatic, transpleural, or hematogeneous metastases (**Fig. 15**) or direct invasion of adjacent primaries. Metastases are rare; direct invasion is more common and results from adjacent pleural or peritoneal malignancies, such as bronchogenic carcinoma or pleural mesothelioma.[11]

The nature and extent of a diaphragmatic mass can be assessed with CT[41]; however, the origin of tumors from the diaphragm or from adjacent tumors may be difficult to determine,[80] and it may also be difficult to confirm whether a tumor is adjacent to or infiltrates the diaphragm. This distinction however may be important in particular for therapeutic planning and assessing the respectability of pleural tumors such as mesotheliomas. Multiplanar reconstructions might be helpful in assessing the diaphragmatic infiltration (**Figs. 16** and **17**).

In summary, the diaphragm is a complex structure that can be assessed directly or indirectly on different imaging modalities. Its position is easily

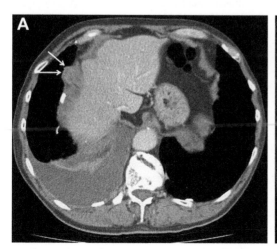
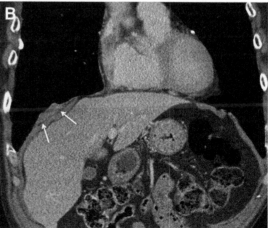

Fig. 17. Contrast-enhanced CT scan of a right-sided metastasizing mesothelioma. Soft tissue nodules are seen along the right diaphragm (*arrows*). On coronal reconstructions, the diaphragm is separated by a fat layer from the pleural metastases, suggesting that the diaphragm is not infiltrated.

appreciated on chest radiographs, but the interpretation of an abnormal position shows a considerable overlap between primary diaphragmatic conditions involving the phrenic nerve, and secondary involvement of the diaphragm from pulmonary and/or abdominal processes. Recently, the direct evaluation of the adjacent organs of the chest (ie, pleura and lungs) and abdomen with ultrasound or CT has replaced the dynamic evaluation of the diaphragmatic motion using fluoroscopy or ultrasound. Imaging of the diaphragm is done intentionally to assess a known or suspected abnormality, but more often it is done unintentionally as the diaphragm is captured on examinations of the chest and abdomen. The complex anatomy of the diaphragm makes complete visualization challenging, but CT and MRI with multiplanar reconstruction are the most useful imaging modalities.

REFERENCES

1. Taylor AM, Jhooti P, Keegan J, et al. Magnetic resonance navigator echo diaphragm monitoring in patients with suspected diaphragm paralysis. J Magn Reson Imaging 1999;9:69–74.

2. Gierada DS, Slone RM, Fleishman MJ. Imaging evaluation of the diaphragm. Chest Surg Clin N Am 1998;8(2):237–80.

3. Diament MJ, Boechat MI, Kangarloo H. Real-time sector ultrasound in the evaluation of suspected abnormalities of diaphragmatic motion. J Clin Ultrasound 1985;13:539–43.

4. Gottesman E, McCool FD. Ultrasound evaluation of the paralyzed diaphragm. Am J Respir Crit Care Med 1997;155:1570–4.

5. Houston JG, Fleet M, Cowan MD, et al. Comparison of ultrasound with fluoroscopy in the assessment of suspected hemidiaphragmatic movement abnormality. Clin Radiol 1995;50:95–8.

6. Juhl JH. Diseases of the pleura, mediastinum, and diaphragm. In: Juhl JH, Crummy AB, editors. Paul and Juhl's essentials of radiologic imaging. 5th edition. Philadelphia: Lippincott; 1987. p. 935–71.

7. Lennon EA, Simon G. The height of the diaphragm in the chest radiograph of normal adults. Br J Radiol 1965;38:937–43.

8. Felson B. Chest roentgenology. Philadelphia: WB Saunders; 1973.

9. Armstrong P. Normal chest. In: Armstrong P, Wilson AG, Dee P, et al, editors. Imaging of diseases of the chest. 2nd edition. St. Louis (MO): Mosby; 1995. p. 15–47.

10. Okuda K, Nomura F, Kawai M, et al. Age related gross changes of the liver and right diaphragm, with special reference to partial eventration. Br J Radiol 1979;52:870–5.

11. Mueller N, Silva IS. Unilateral elevation of the diaphragm. Imaging consult, Available at: http://imaging.consult.com. Accessed March 25, 2009. St. Louis (MO): Elsevier; 2008.

12. Tarver RD, Conces DJJ, Cory DA, et al. Imaging the diaphragm and its disorders. J Thorac Imaging 1989;4:1–18.

13. Vogl A, Small A. Partial eventration of the right diaphragm (congenital diaphragmatic herniation of liver). Ann Intern Med 1955;43:61–82.

14. Hesselink JR, Chung KJ, Peters ME, et al. Congenital partial eventration of the left diaphragm. Am J Roentgenol 1978;131:417–9.

15. Celli BR. Respiratory management of diaphragm paralysis. Semin Respir Crit Care Med 2002;23:275–81.

16. Blair E, Hickam JB. The effect of change in body position on lung volume and intrapulmonary gas mixing in normal subjects. J Clin Invest 1955;34:383–9.

17. Fraser RS, Pare JAP, Fraser RG, et al. Synopsis of diseases of the chest. 2nd edition. Philadelphia: WB Saunders; 1994.

18. Kawashima A, Libshitz HI. Malignant pleural mesothelioma: CT manifestations in 50 cases. Am J Roentgenol 1990;155:965–9.

19. Rabinowitz JG, Efremidis SC, Cohen B, et al. A comparative study of mesothelioma and asbestosis using computed tomography and conventional chest radiography. Radiology 1982;144:453–60.

20. Alexander C. Diaphragm movements and the diagnosis of diaphragmatic paralysis. Clin Radiol 1966;17:79–83.

21. Gierada DS, Curtin JJ, Erickson SJ, et al. Diaphragmatic motion: fast gradient recalled-echo MR imaging in healthy subjects. Radiology 1995;194:879–84.

22. Harris RS, Giovanetti M, Kim BK. Normal ventilatory movement of the right hemidiaphragm studied by ultrasonography and pneumotachography. Radiology 1983;146:141–4.

23. Houston JG, Morris AD, Howie CA, et al. Technical report: quantitative assessment of diaphragmatic movement—a reproducible method using ultrasound. Clin Radiol 1992;46:405–7.

24. Simon G, Bonnell J, Kazantzis G, et al. Some radiological observations on the range of movement of the diaphragm. Clin Radiol 1969;20:231–3.

25. Loh L, Goldman M, Davis JN. The assessment of diaphragmatic function. Medicine 1977;56:165–9.

26. Arborelius M, Lilja B, Senyk J. Regional and total lung function studies in patients with hemidiaphragmatic paralysis. Respiration 1975;32:253–64.

27. Roussos C, Macklem PT. The respiratory muscles. N Engl J Med 1982;307:786–97.

28. Piehler JM, Pairolero PC, Gracey DR, et al. Unexplained diaphragmatic paralysis: a harbinger of malignant disease? J Thorac Cardiovasc Surg 1982;84:861–4.

29. Higgenbottam T, Allen D, Loh L, et al. Abdominal wall movement in normals and in patients with hemidiaphragmatic and bilateral diaphragmatic palsy. Thorax 1977;32:589–95.

30. Ch'en IY, Armstrong JD II. Value of fluoroscopy in patients with suspected bilateral hemidiaphragmatic paralysis. AJR Am J Roentgenol 1993;160:29–31.

31. Dietrich P, Alsofrom G. The diaphragm. In: Taveras JM, Ferrucci JT, editors. Radiology: Diagonosis, Imaging, Intervation. Philadelphia: Lippincott; 1990. p. 1–10.

32. Derenne JPH, Macklem PT, Roussos CH. The respiratory muscles: mechanics, control, and pathophysiology. Am Rev Respir Dis 1978;118:581–601.

33. Rigatto M, DeMedeiros NP. Diaphragmatic flutter: report of a case and review of literature. Am J Med 1962;132:103–9.

34. Eren S, Ciris F. Diaphragmatic hernia: diagnostic approaches with review of the literature. Eur J Radiol 2005;54:448–59.

35. Caskey CI, Zerhouni EA, Fishman EK, et al. Aging of the diaphragm: a CT study. Radiology 1989;171:385–9.

36. Pearson FG, Cooper JD, Ilves R, et al. Massive hiatal hernia with incarceration: a report of 53 cases. Ann Thorac Surg 1983;35:45–51.

37. Vanamo K. A 45-year perspective of congenital diaphragmatic hernia. Br J Surg 1996;83:1758–62.

38. Gale ME. Bochdalek hernia: prevalence and CT characteristics. Radiology 1985;156:449–52.

39. Mullins ME, Stein J, Saini SS, et al. Prevalence of incidental Bochdalek's hernia in a large adult population. AJR Am J Roentgenol 2001;177:363–6.

40. Raymond GS, Miller RM, Müller NL, et al. Congenital thoracic lesions that mimic neoplastic disease on chest radiographs of adults. AJR Am J Roentgenol 1997;168:763–9.

41. Yamana D, Ohba S. Three-dimensional image of Bochdalek diaphragmatic hernia: a case report. Radiat Med 1994;12:39–41.

42. Panicek DM, Benson CB, Gottlieb RH, et al. The diaphragm: anatomic, pathologic, and radiologic considerations. Radiographics 1988;8:385–425.

43. Wallace DB. Intrapericardial diaphragmatic hernia. Radiology 1977;122:596.

44. Gaerte SC, Meyer CA, Winer-Muram HT, et al. Fat-containing lesions of the chest. Radiographics 2002;22:S61–78.

45. LaRosa DV, Esham RH, Morgan SL, et al. Diaphragmatic hernia of Morgagni. Southampt Med J 1999;92:409–11.

46. Shah R, Sabanathan S, Mearns AJ, et al. Traumatic rupture of diaphragm. Ann Thorac Surg 1995;60:1444–9.

47. Gelman R, Mirvis SE, Gens D. Diaphragmatic rupture due to blunt trauma: sensitivity of plain chest radiographs. AJR Am J Roentgenol 1991;156:51–7.

48. Shackleton KL, Stewart ET, Taylor AJ. Traumatic diaphragmatic injuries: spectrum of radiographic findings. Radiographics 1998;18:49–59.

49. Symbas PN. Blunt traumatic rupture of the diaphragm. Ann Thorac Surg 1978;26:193–4.

50. Perlman SJ, Rogers LF, Mintzer RA, et al. Abnormal course of nasogastric tube in traumatic rupture of left hemidiaphragm. AJR Am J Roentgenol 1984;142:85–6.

51. Hegarty MM, Bryer JV, Angorn IB, et al. Delayed presentation of traumatic diaphragmatic hernia. Ann Surg 1978;188:229–33.

52. Heiberg E, Wolverson MK, Hurd RN, et al. CT recognition of traumatic rupture of the diaphragm. AJR Am J Roentgenol 1980;135:369–72.

53. Gourin A, Garzow AA. Diagnostic problems in traumatic diaphragmatic hernia. J Trauma 1974;14:20–31.

54. Guth AA, Pachter HL, Kim U. Pitfalls in the diagnosis of blunt diaphragmatic injury. Am J Surg 1995;170:5–9.

55. Rodriguez-Morales G, Rodriguez A, Shatney CH. Acute rupture of the diaphragm in blunt trauma: analysis of 60 patients. J Trauma 1986;26:438–44.

56. Voeller GR, Reisser JR, Fabian TC, et al. Blunt diaphragm injuries. A five-year experience. Am Surg 1990;56:28–31.

57. Ward RE, Flynn TC, Clark WP. Diaphragmatic disruption secondary to blunt abdominal trauma. J Trauma 1981;21:35–8.

58. Estrera AS, Platt MR, Mills LT. Traumatic injuries of the diaphragm. Chest 1979;75:306–13.

59. Ball T, McCrory R, Smith JO, et al. Traumatic diaphragmatic hernia: errors in diagnosis. AJR Am J Roentgenol 1982;138:633–7.

60. Bekassy SM, Dave KS, Wooler GH, et al. 'Spontaneous' and traumatic rupture of the diaphragm. Ann Surg 1973;177:320–4.

61. Ammann AM, Brewer WH, Maull KI, et al. Truamatic rupture of the diaphragm: real time sonographic diagnosis. AJR Am J Roentgenol 1983;140:915–6.

62. Payne JH, Yellin AE. Traumatic diaphragmatic hernia. Arch Surg 1982;117:18–24.

63. Bergin D, Ennis R, Keogh C, et al. The "dependent viscera" sign in CT diagnosis of blunt traumatic diaphragmatic rupture. AJR Am J Roentgenol 2001;177:1137–40.

64. Murray JG, Caoili E, Gruden JF, et al. Acute rupture of the diaphragm due to blunt trauma: diagnostic sensitivity and specificity of CT. AJR Am J Roentgenol 1996;166:1035–9.

65. Worthy SA, Kang EY, Hartman TE, et al. Diaphragmatic rupture: CT findings in 11 patients. Radiology 1995;194:885–8.

66. Demos TC, Soloman C, Posniak HV, et al. Computed tomography in traumatic defects of the diaphragm. Clin Imaging 1989;13:62–7.

67. Holland DG, Quint LE. Traumatic rupture of the diaphragm without visceral herniation: CT diagnosis. AJR Am J Roentgenol 1991;157:17–8.

68. Israel RS, Mayberry JC, Primack SL. Diaphragmatic rupture: use of helical CT scanning with multiplanar reformations. AJR Am J Roentgenol 1996;167: 1201–3.

69. Gale ME. Anterior diaphragm: variations in the CT appearance. Radiology 1986;161:635–9.

70. Kleinmann PK, Raptopoulos V. The anterior diaphragmatic attachments: an anatomic and radiologic study with clinical correlates. Radiology 1985; 155:289–93.

71. Anda S, Roysland P, Fougner R, et al. CT appearance of the diaphragm varying with respiratory phase and muscular tension. J Comput Assist Tomogr 1986;10:744–5.

72. Rosen A, Auh YH, Rubenstein WA, et al. CT appearance of diaphragmatic pseudotumors. J Comput Assist Tomogr 1983;7:995–9.

73. Williamson BRJ, Gouse JC, Rohrer DG, et al. Variation in the thickness of the diaphragmatic crura with respiration. Radiology 1987;163:683–4.

74. Brink JA, Heiken JP, Semenkovich J, et al. Abnormalities of the diaphragm and adjacent structures: findings on multiplanar spiral CT scans. AJR Am J Roentgenol 1994;163:307–10.

75. Gierada DS, Curtin JJ, Erickson SJ, et al. Fast gradient echo magnetic resonance imaging of the normal diaphragm. J Thorac Imaging 1996;12:70–4.

76. Anderson LS, Forrest JV. Tumors of the diaphragm. Am J Roentgenol Radium Ther Nucl Med 1973; 119:259–65.

77. Olafsson G, Rausing A, Holen O. Primary tumors of the diaphragm. Chest 1971;59:568–70.

78. Ferguson DD, Westcott JL. Lipoma of the diaphragm. Report of a case. Radiology 1976;118: 527–8.

79. Tihansky DP, Lopez GM. Bilateral lipomas of the diaphragm. N Y State J Med 1988;88:151–2.

80. Schwartz EE, Wechsler RJ. Diaphragmatic and paradia-phragmatic tumors and pseudotumors. J Thorac Imaging 1989;4:19–28.

81. Castillo M, Shirkhoda A. Computed tomography of diaphragmatic lipoma. J Comput Assist Tomogr 1985;9:167–70.

Surgical Conditions of the Diaphragm: Posterior Diaphragmatic Hernias in Infants

Priscilla P.L. Chiu, MD, PhD, Jacob C. Langer, MD*

KEYWORDS

- Congenital diaphragmatic hernia
- Extracorporeal membrane oxygenation
- Gentle ventilation • Pulmonary hypoplasia
- Pulmonary hypertension • Morbidity

Congenital diaphragmatic hernia (CDH) is a defect of the diaphragm associated with herniation of abdominal viscera into the chest cavity. Related conditions of the diaphragm that mimic CDH but are not associated with diaphragmatic defects include diaphragmatic eventration and phrenic nerve palsy. These two conditions result in a mechanically impaired "high-riding" diaphragm without visceral herniation. The locations of the defect in CDH include posterolateral defect (foramen of Bochdalek), anterior/retrosternal defect (foramen of Morgagni), crural defect (para-esophageal hernia), and diaphragmatic agenesis (**Fig. 1**). Of these, Bochdalek CDH and agenesis are the most common and are associated with the greatest complexity and mortality risk.[1] In this article, we focus on the diagnosis and management of these two related entities.

EMBRYOLOGY

The diaphragm starts to form during the fourth week of embryological development from four components of mesodermal structures. Lateral extension of the septum transversum from the midline joining to the lateral margins of the pleuroperitoneal fold results in the formation of the membranous (central tendon) and muscular diaphragm (**Fig. 2**). The esophageal mesentery extends into the pleuroperitoneal fold to form the crural and dorsal portions of the diaphragm. Abdominal wall-derived mesenchyme migrates inward to fuse with the other components. Finally, lung expansion is thought to promote the fusion of all layers, resulting in a single fibromuscular tissue that physically separates the thoracic and abdominal cavities by the end of the 12th week.[2]

Diaphragmatic defects are thought to result from the failure of one or more of these layers to fuse with each other. In the case of Bochdalek hernias, abnormal development of the pleuroperitoneal fold (muscular diaphragm) is thought to result in the typical posterolateral defect as demonstrated through animal models of CDH.[3] Because the right pleuroperitoneal fold is thought to close first, left-sided Bochdalek hernias occur more frequently than right-sided CDH. The most severe CDH cases include complete diaphragmatic agenesis (ie, the complete absence of a muscular diaphragm) and bilateral CDH. The embryological defects associated with the development of anterior or foramen of Morgagni hernias

The authors have no conflicts of interest to declare in the submission of this manuscript for publication. All studies performed by the authors in this report were conducted with institutional ethics board approval.
Division of Pediatric General and Thoracic Surgery, The Hospital for Sick Children, 555 University Avenue, Toronto, ON, Canada M5G 1X8
* Corresponding author.
E-mail address: jacob.langer@sickkids.ca (J.C. Langer).

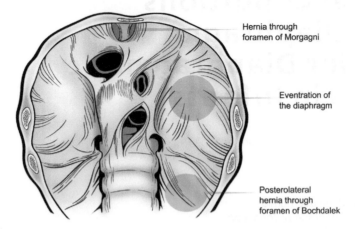

Fig. 1. Types of CDH.

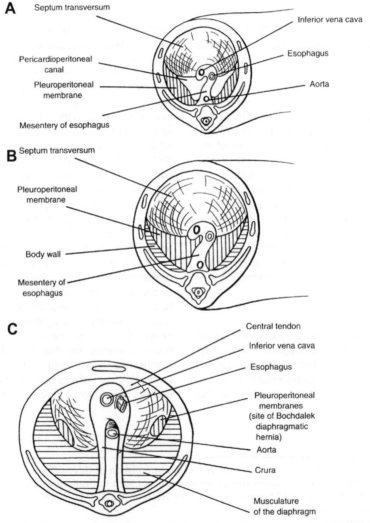

Fig. 2. Embryology of the diaphragm. (*From* Langer JC. Normal fetal development. In: Oldham KT, Colombani PM, Foglia RP, editors. Surgery of infants and children. Philadelphia: Lippincott-Raven Publishers; 1997. p. 44; with permission.)

are less well understood, although it is thought that the retrosternal space exists because of the superior epigastric vessels.[4]

HISTORICAL PERSPECTIVE

Congenital diaphragmatic hernia was first described by the French physician Lazarus Riverius in 1679,[5] and the first pediatric case was described by Sir Charles Holt in 1701.[6] The first surgical repair in a child was reported by O'Dwyer in 1890,[7] and the first neonatal repair was done by Gross in 1946.[8] In 1953, Gross[9] reported an 89% survival rate in 72 patients. Subsequent reports in the 1950s and 1960s documented a decreasing survival rate, and by the late 1970s and early 1980s, reported mortality rates were approximately 50%.[10] This decrease in reported survival rates presumably stemmed from improvements in neonatal resuscitation and transportation, resulting in fewer delivery room deaths and more infants surviving to reach the pediatric surgeon.

In the 1980s, prenatal diagnosis of CDH became possible because of the advent of high-resolution ultrasound, which in many cases led to maternal transport to a perinatal center prior to delivery. Prenatal diagnosis led to inclusion of a higher-risk group of fetuses and newborns in survival reports (the so-called "hidden mortality")[11]; thus, reported survival rates in the early 1990s have been approximately 40%.[12]

CLINICAL FEATURES

The presence of bowel loops within the thorax can be detected on routine antenatal ultrasound or MRI during the second trimester of pregnancy, making possible antenatal diagnosis of the CDH infant in many cases. Radiological indices obtained from antenatal imaging studies, such as polyhydramnios, lung volume, lung/head ratio, and positioning of the left lobe of the liver ("up" in the chest or "down" in the abdominal cavity), have been used to prognosticate the severity of the pulmonary hypoplasia and postnatal mortality risk.[13] In general, worse prognosis is associated with liver-up positioning or when the lung/head ratio is less than 1.4 between 22 and 27 weeks' gestation.[13] In most centers, antenatal diagnosis of CDH should be followed by prenatal counseling and planned term delivery at a high-risk obstetrical unit. The indications for fetal intervention and the efficacy of these interventions remain controversial (see below). In general, term delivery of the CDH infant is preferred and associated with the best outcomes.[14]

Despite the increase in antenatally diagnosed CDH cases, many infants still present postnatally without prenatal diagnosis. In most cases, the CDH neonate typically presents with variable degrees of respiratory distress, absent or decreased breath sounds on the affected side, and a scaphoid abdomen. Often, the chest radiograph shows mediastinal shift. In the case of a left-sided CDH, the presence of gas-filled bowel loops and a nasogastric tube in the left chest are diagnostic for a left CDH (**Fig. 3**). Right-sided CDH may be associated with more subtle changes on chest radiograph, as liver herniation may not be suspected on routine radiograph unless associated with herniated bowel loops (**Fig. 4**). In addition to radiographs, other modalities for confirming the presence of CDH include ultrasound, and intestinal contrast studies to detect the presence of herniated organs within the chest.

Rarely, CDH presents late in infancy, later in childhood, or even in adulthood. This delay in presentation is due to the small size of the diaphragmatic defect with asymptomatic herniation of abdominal viscera. Such delayed presentations are rarely associated with any cardiorespiratory compromise but can present a significant risk if the abdominal viscera become incarcerated through the small diaphragmatic defect, resulting in gastric or intestinal strangulation, sepsis, short bowel syndrome, or death (**Fig. 5**).[15]

INCIDENCE AND PATHOPHYSIOLOGY

The incidence of CDH is approximately 1 in 4000 live births, although the population incidence is slightly higher.[16] Left-sided CDH is more common (80% of cases) compared to right-sided CDH (20%), but right-sided CDH is reported to have a greater mortality risk.[17] The major causes of

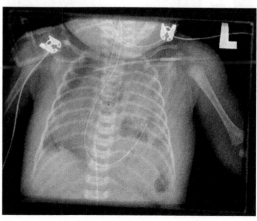

Fig. 3. Left-sided CDH on chest radiograph.

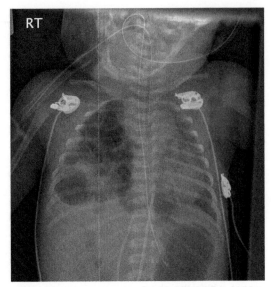

Fig. 4. Right-sided CDH on chest radiograph.

mortality in infants with CDH are pulmonary hypo-plasia, pulmonary hypertension, and associated congenital anomalies, especially cardiac defects.

Associated Anomalies

Most commonly, CDH presents as an isolated defect; however, approximately 10% of CDH infants may present at birth with other anomalies, including cardiac, urogenital, brain, or spinal cord defects. Genetic syndromes associated with CDH include trisomy 13, 18, and 21; Fryns syndrome; Cornelia de Lange syndrome; Denys-Drash syndrome; and Donnai-Barrow syndrome.[18] Potentially lethal structural or chromosomal anom-alies are found in 30% to 40% of CDH infants in population-based studies,[19] although reports that

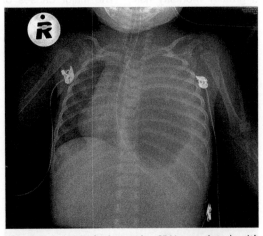

Fig. 5. Incarcerated viscera in CDH associated with respiratory failure.

include both antenatal and postnatal data have cited rates of potentially lethal anomalies at 50%.[18]

Pulmonary Hypoplasia

Most infants with CDH have pulmonary hypoplasia, which results in a variable degree of respiratory insufficiency.[20] The hypoplastic lung consists of fewer branch airways with relative paucity of alve-olar terminal structures compared to normal lung tissue.[21] Although the exact etiology is unclear, pulmonary hypoplasia is traditionally thought to result from compression of the developing lung by the herniated viscera, which may even contribute to hypoplasia of the contralateral lung if mediastinal shift is present.[22] This theory is consistent with observations that CDH identified later in gestation is associated with lower mortality[23] and, in animal models, with a thoracic space–occupying mass or a diaphragmatic defect that results in pulmonary hypoplasia.[24] However, data from teratogen-induced models of CDH suggest that pulmonary hypoplasia occurs before or simultaneous with the development of the diaphragmatic defect,[25] suggesting a common developmental pathway affecting both lung and diaphragm development rather than a "cause-and-effect" relationship.[26] This theory is supported by observations of Fryns syndrome patients who have pulmonary hypo-plasia with or without CDH defect.[27] Finally, the "dual-hit" hypothesis integrates both theories about pulmonary hypoplasia observed in the nitro-fen model for CDH.[28]

Pulmonary Hypertension

Pulmonary hypertension in CDH infants results from the decreased number of pulmonary arterial struc-tures associated with overmuscularization of the terminal vessels of the hypoplastic lung[21] and failure of postnatal remodeling,[29] resulting in increased right heart resistance, perfusion bias to the unaf-fected side, and increased shunting. Clinically, pulmonary hypertension presents after a "honey-moon period" during the first 12 to 24 hours of life, where the initial stability is replaced by right-to-left shunting (either through the patent ductus arterio-sus, foramen ovale, or other endocardial cushion defects), resulting in hypoxia and hypercarbia. Recalcitrant pulmonary hypertension remains a leading cause of mortality for CDH patients.

MANAGEMENT OF THE CRITICALLY ILL NEONATE WITH CONGENITAL DIAPHRAGMATIC HERNIA

The ongoing challenge to CDH survival remains the optimal management of the underlying pulmonary hypoplasia and pulmonary hypertension. Therefore, the priorities of current CDH management are to support respiratory function using lung preservation strategies and to achieve hemodynamic stability to minimize overall morbidity.

Initial Resuscitation

The immediate management of a CDH neonate consists of respiratory monitoring, insertion of nasogastric tube for bowel decompression, establishment of intravenous access, and application of oxygen by noninvasive means or, if respiratory compromise is apparent, by invasive endotracheal intubation. Use of noninvasive positive-pressure respiratory support (ie, nasal or bag-mask continuous positive airway pressure) should be avoided because it leads to further gaseous distension of the herniated viscera, which may further exacerbate cardiorespiratory compromise. In those CDH patients who display minimal signs of respiratory distress, routine imaging and laboratory investigations before elective CDH repair are the only investigations required. More commonly, CDH patients present with gross respiratory failure requiring immediate endotracheal intubation, fluid resuscitation, and hemodynamic support. The most common tools used to support the most severely affected CDH neonates are "gentle ventilation" techniques, extracorporeal membrane oxygenation (ECMO), and pulmonary vasodilators. Surgical repair of the CDH is generally deferred until the infant is stabilized.

Ventilator Management

It is now recognized that high-pressure mechanical ventilation results in ventilator-induced lung damage, which ultimately causes neonatal respiratory failure and death, or, in CDH survivors, iatrogenic bronchopulmonary dysplasia.[30] To preserve and protect lung function in the context of CDH-related pulmonary hypoplasia, the gentle ventilation approach uses a minimal ventilatory strategy of permissive hypercapnea while maintaining an acceptable level of oxygenation and ventilation through conventional or high-frequency oscillation ventilation techniques.[20] Positive end expiratory pressure is restricted to 5 cm H_2O to minimize barotrauma to the hypoplastic lung. High-frequency oscillation ventilation is now routinely used early to gently ventilate the CDH patient when ventilatory pressures creep up as the oxygenation levels decrease. Once ventilation stabilizes, the patient is weaned back to conventional ventilation. Operative repair can be performed either when the patient is weaned back to conventional ventilation or while on high-frequency oscillation ventilation.

Extracorporeal Membrane Oxygenation

Since ECMO was first shown to be beneficial to the CDH population, multiple series have reported improved survival using ECMO support for lung preservation when standard therapies have failed.[31,32] Initially, ECMO was used to support CDH infants postoperatively.[33] With the trend towards delayed CDH repair in the early 1990s, ECMO became more commonly used as part of preoperative stabilization[34] and subsequent repair on ECMO,[35] particularly among high-risk infants.[36] However, this was associated with a higher risk of bleeding, sepsis, and other complications,[37] leading some to advocate delaying repair until the patient has been weaned off of ECMO support.[38]

The primary role of ECMO is to provide respiratory support during the early postnatal period of pulmonary vascular reactivity. As pulmonary hypoplasia remains the leading cause of death of CDH patients on ECMO, it is clear that ECMO does not reverse the underlying pulmonary defect in CDH and that its use may be futile in patients with lethal pulmonary hypoplasia (ie, those who have never demonstrated normal Pao_2 levels).[39] In many centers, ventilatory criteria for ECMO cannulation include the inability to maintain preductal oxygen saturations greater than 85%; peak inspiratory pressure greater than 28 cm H_2O or mean airway pressure greater than 15 cm H_2O; pressure-resistant hypotension; inadequate oxygen delivery based on persistent metabolic acidosis or rising serum lactate level; and inability to wean from fraction of inspired oxygen (Fio_2) 100% in the first 48 hours of life. When the patient requires more than the set level of ventilatory support, clinicians use ECMO rather than escalate the settings on positive-pressure ventilation. Other inclusion criteria include birth weight greater than 2 kg, gestational age over 34 weeks, absence of intracranial hemorrhage greater than grade I, and absence of other congenital or chromosomal anomalies.[32]

Pulmonary Hypertension Management

The management of pulmonary hypertension in CDH infants remains a challenge. Pulse oximetry monitoring can reveal preductal and postductal arterial oxygen saturation gradients, indicating the persistence of right-to-left shunting through a patent ductus arteriosus or septal defect. In cases of severe pulmonary hypertension, the patent ductus arteriosus serves as a "pressure release" valve and preserves cardiac output and right heart function.[20] Two-dimensional echocardiography remains the best modality for the real-time assessment and monitoring of pulmonary arterial pressure and right heart function at the bedside.[40] In the presence of high right ventricular pressures or decreased right ventricular function, adjunctive treatments are required to control pulmonary hypertension prior to surgical repair.

The utility of pharmacologic pulmonary vasodilators, such as inhaled nitric oxide, sildenafil (a type 5 phosphodiesterase inhibitor), prostacyclines, and bosentan (an endothelin-1 receptor antagonist), remains speculative for CDH patients as no studies have shown significant benefits in the treatment of CDH-associated pulmonary hypertension. Results from the largest randomized, controlled trial of early inhaled nitric oxide therapy in patients with CDH failed to show any difference in the combined end point of death/ECMO-use between controls and patients treated with inhaled nitric oxide.[41] Despite the lack of clear evidence, however, inhaled nitric oxide is widely used in this group of patients.

The use of ECMO to stabilize recalcitrant pulmonary hypertension with or without concomitant ventilatory compromise remains an option,[42] but the static component of pulmonary hypertension may be insurmountable if pulmonary hypoplasia is severe. Weaning a patient from ECMO support in this scenario is often difficult in conjunction with associated respiratory failure, and the mortality risk for this patient population is high.[13]

Surgical Repair and Timing

It was previously thought that early CDH repair was critical to achieve respiratory stabilization because herniated contents had to be reduced to decrease intrathoracic pressures and because two intact diaphragms were needed to improve respiratory mechanics.[43,44] However, the stress of operative repair can result in further respiratory deterioration and instability secondary to a decrease in pulmonary compliance in the fragile CDH neonate.[30] Therefore, surgical repair for the unstable patient is now deferred until cardiorespiratory stabilization is achieved.[43,44]

The fundamental objectives of CDH surgical treatment are the reduction of the herniated contents and closure of the diaphragmatic defect either primarily, if the defect is small, or with a patch, for larger defects. The conventional approach to CDH repair is via the abdomen through a subcostal incision. Small diaphragmatic defects can be closed using with nonabsorbable, interrupted sutures. Large CDH defects require

either an abdominal wall muscle flap[45] or a synthetic patch (**Fig. 6**). The "ideal" patch material remains elusive. Current patch repair materials include engineered biosynthetic porcine submucosal matrix, Marlex, polytetrafluoroethylene (PTFE), and porcine dermis.[46] CDH patients requiring patch repair have increased morbidity and mortality rates compared to those repaired without a patch,[47,48] which like reflects not the type of repair but rather the greater instability (eg, patch repair on ECMO)[49] or more severe underlying pulmonary defects (eg, complete diaphragmatic agenesis) associated with these CDH patients.[50] Additionally, CDH patients requiring prosthetic patch repair have greater long-term morbidity, including increased incidence of patch infection, bowel obstruction, diaphragmatic hernia recurrence, and development of chest and abdominal wall deformities.[47]

Recently, minimal access surgery techniques using laparoscopic[51,52] or thoracoscopic[53,54] approaches (**Fig. 7**) to CDH repair have been reported in relatively stable newborns, as well as in older children with CDH. The apparent advantages of small incisions, better cosmetic results, less postoperative pain, and possibly fewer long-term musculoskeletal sequelae compared to the conventional abdominal incision have made minimal access surgery repair an attractive option. While early results indicate that this approach is technically feasible and safe, data on long-term outcomes are lacking.

The routine use of chest tubes to drain the affected pleural cavity has largely been abandoned as chest drainage may promote infectious contamination of the pleural space without the benefit of accelerating ipsilateral lung expansion postrepair.[44] Rarely, a "tension" pleural effusion, usually chylous, may develop, resulting in impaired pulmonary function and ventilation, necessitating the insertion of a chest tube.[55] The frequency of

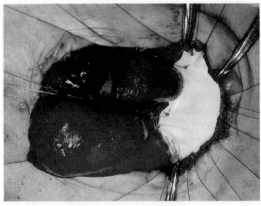

Fig. 6. Synthetic patch repair of CDH.

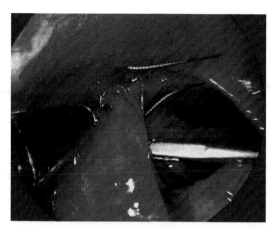

Fig. 7. Thoracoscopic repair of CDH.

postrepair pneumothorax has decreased with the use of pressure-limited ventilation, decreasing the incidence rate from 25%[30] to less than 5%.[56]

A large proportion of patients who are stabilized on ECMO preoperatively undergo repair while on ECMO.[34] Recent reports indicate that, of the patients placed on ECMO prerepair, the majority underwent repair while on ECMO, while roughly one third underwent repair post-decannulation, leaving 16% that were never repaired.[57–59] Infants who underwent repair on ECMO had a 50% mortality rate. The greatest risk of CDH repair on ECMO is hemorrhage,[35,60] with aminocaproic acid (Amicar), an inhibitor of fibrinolysis, now widely used to minimize hemorrhage risks during repair.[61,62]

Surfactant Replacement

Pulmonary insufficiency is thought to be exacerbated by surfactant deficiency in both human and animal models of CDH.[63] However, surfactant replacement therapy has not been shown to improve patient survival in term,[64] preterm,[65] or ECMO-treated[66] CDH patients. In fact, there is evidence that this treatment may harm rather than help the CDH infant.[64]

Fetal Surgery

Antenatal herniation of abdominal viscera into the thorax can result in significant mediastinal shift, impaired cardiac output, fetal distress, and fetal hydrops. Because of the presence of fluid in the chest cavity and other signs of fetal distress, fetal ultrasound or MRI can detect these changes. In cases where fetal demise appears imminent, preterm delivery and early CDH repair may seem an attractive option, but the resultant prematurity may further complicate the postnatal course for the CDH infant. In some centers, prenatal drainage

(via insertion of an amniothoracic shunt) of the pleural effusion associated with the CDH may help relieve the mediastinal shift, restore cardiac output, and alleviate fetal distress to allow for term and near-term delivery via cesarean section.[67]

Animal studies from the 1980s suggested that in utero repair of CDH might lead to lung growth and an improvement in survival.[68] However, significant intraoperative mortality and preterm delivery after maternal hysterotomy made experience with human CDH repair disappointing.[69,70] Subsequent recognition in experimental studies that tracheal obstruction in animal models of CDH resulted in accelerated lung growth[71,72] led to the development of a number of techniques to occlude the fetal trachea in humans with CDH. Although initial procedures were done using open hysterotomy,[71] minimal access surgery techniques were ultimately developed using single-port fetoscopy.[73,74]

The only randomized control study of fetal tracheal occlusion for CDH patients failed to demonstrate a significant difference in outcomes compared to the control patient group.[75] Despite the findings of this study, there is continuing interest in antenatal intervention using ultrasound-guided and fetoscopic balloon occlusion of the trachea to "correct" the pulmonary hypoplasia associated with CDH.[76] However, there is currently insufficient evidence to verify the benefit or substantiate the broad application of this or any other fetal intervention in the current management of CDH.

Liquid Ventilation

Liquid ventilation has been tested experimentally and clinically for the management of respiratory failure due to surfactant deficiency. Among the many benefits of liquid ventilation, both total liquid ventilation and partial liquid ventilation, are improved gas exchange by lowering alveolar surface tension and improving lung compliance, resulting in lower ventilation pressures and less ventilator-induced lung injury.[77] These benefits make liquid ventilation an attractive option for CDH infants. Despite initial studies in CDH animal models and human subjects showing improved gas exchange[78,79] and accelerated lung growth,[80,81] a multicenter study examining the use of partial liquid ventilation in CDH respiratory failure ended prematurely, because of the small number of enrolled subjects, with a failure to demonstrate any improvement.[82]

Lung Transplantation

There are few reports in the literature on lung transplantation for CDH, but it remains a final option for those CDH infants with refractory and life-threatening pulmonary hypoplasia and pulmonary hypertension.[83,84] The main limitations to lung transplantation for the CDH neonate are timely availability of donor lungs, scarcity of size-matched lungs or lobes for the infant chest, and maintenance of cardiorespiratory stability of the sick CDH infant with bridging technologies, such as ECMO, that could render the patient ineligible for transplantation (eg, severe intracranial hemorrhage). The paucity of experience with neonatal lung transplantation would suggest that this treatment option remains experimental for CDH infants.

LONG-TERM OUTCOME

The use of lung preservation strategies in the past decade has been accompanied by a remarkable improvement in CDH survival. The international literature has reported increases in CDH survival from 50% in the mid-1990s[85,86] to the current 80% to 90% survival to discharge.[87,88] Given the significant improvements in patient survival achieved over the past decades, the focus in CDH management has shifted to the minimization of survivor morbidity. Recent CDH survivors have a higher incidence of respiratory, nutritional, musculoskeletal, neurodevelopmental, and gastrointestinal morbidity compared to historical cohorts,[89–91] although most of these conditions appear to improve with patient growth. The exception is chest wall deformity, which become more apparent, especially during adolescence.[90]

With the use of lung preservation strategies, there has been a decrease in iatrogenic lung damage with resultant bronchopulmonary dysplasia among CDH survivors. However, the underlying pulmonary hypoplasia persists and some CDH survivors continue to experience cardiorespiratory compromise as demonstrated by persistent tachypnea, oxygen dependence, and failure to thrive in early childhood. These patients often require feeding tubes for nutritional supplementation as their tachypnea renders them poor oral feeders and limits their ability to take sufficient calories to maintain their growth. Home oxygen therapy is necessary for some CDH patients with persistent hypoxia and pulmonary hypertension. The frailest of CDH patients with prolonged intensive care unit stay often have multiple neurological deficits and require occupational and physiotherapy to help their transition from the acute care setting to home.

Gastroesophageal reflux is very common among CDH survivors, with 40% to 50% of survivors affected.[89,90] The sequelae of ongoing reflux in CDH patients include failure to thrive,

aspiration pneumonia, and respiratory compromise. Although many can be medically managed, those with severe pulmonary hypoplasia and large CDH defects requiring patch repairs are most likely to require surgical management with fundoplication.[92,93]

Neurodevelopmental deficits are not infrequent among CDH survivors, as 15% to 20% of patients demonstrate neurological or neuromuscular impairment due to the use of ECMO, muscle relaxants, and ototoxic drugs during acute management.[94,95] Many recent reports have consistently documented the high incidence of hearing loss among CDH survivors and the long-term requirement for hearing-assist devices.[90,96]

Although signs of chest wall deformities following CDH repair may be evident in early childhood, more long-term follow-up data are required to reveal the true incidence of musculoskeletal effects of CDH repair, especially as these changes become more apparent during adolescence,[90] indicating the need for long-term follow-up of CDH survivors well beyond their early childhood years. Many institutions have formed multidisciplinary follow-up clinics to properly monitor the multisystem morbidity that CDH patients may develop.[59]

SUMMARY

The care of the neonate with CDH has significantly evolved from an approach characterized by aggressive ventilation and emergency surgical repair, to the current use of permissive hypercapnea, physiologic stabilization, elective surgical repair, and multidisciplinary follow-up. Overall survival now approaches 80%, but this improvement has been associated with increased recognition of respiratory, cardiac, gastrointestinal, and neurodevelopmental morbidity. Topics of continuing controversy in the management of CDH include the value of fetal tracheal occlusion, the expanding role of ECMO, and the use of minimal access techniques for surgical repair.

REFERENCES

1. Lally KP, Lally PA, Van Meurs KP, et al. Treatment evolution in high-risk congenital diaphragmatic hernia. Ten years' experience with diaphragmatic agenesis. Ann Surg 2006;244(4):505–13.

2. Skandalakis JE, Gray SW, Ricketts RR. The diaphragm. In: Skandalakis JE, Gray SW, editors. Embryology for surgeons, vol. 1. Baltimore (MD): Williams & Wilkins; 1994. p. 491–539.

3. Clugston RD, Greer JJ. Diaphragm development and congenital diaphragmatic hernia. Semin Pediatr Surg 2007;16:94–100.

4. Moore KL, Persaud T. The developing human: clinically oriented embryology, vol. 1. Philadelphia: WB Saunders; 1993. p. 174–85.

5. Puri P, Wester T. Historical aspects of congenital diaphragmatic hernia. Pediatr Surg Int 1997;12:95–100.

6. Holt CA. Child who had its intestines, mesentery, &c in the cavity of the thorax, and a further account of the person mentioned to have swallowed stones, in No. 253 of these transactions. Phil Trans 1700–1701;22:992–4.

7. Irish M, Holm B, Glick P. Congenital diaphragmatic hernia: a historical review. Clin Perinatol 1996;23(4):625–53.

8. Gross R. Congenital hernia of the diaphragm. Am J Dis Child 1946;71:579–92.

9. Gross R. Congenital hernia of the diaphragm. The surgery of infancy and childhood. Philadelphia: W.B. Saunders Company; 1953. p. 428–44.

10. Reynolds M, Luck SR, Lappen R. The "critical" neonate with diaphragmatic hernia: a 21-year perspective. J Pediatr Surg 1984;19(4):364–9.

11. Harrison M, Bjordal R, Langmark F, et al. Congenital diaphragmatic hernia: the hidden mortality. J Pediatr Surg 1978;13(3):227–30.

12. Harrison M, Adzick N, Estes J, et al. A prospective study of the outcome for fetuses with diaphragmatic hernia. J Am Med Assoc 1994;271(5):382–4.

13. Hedrick HL, Danzer E, Merchant A, et al. Liver position and lung-to-head ratio for prediction of extracorporeal membrane oxygenation and survival in isolated left congenital diaphragmatic hernia. Am J Obstet Gynecol 2007;197(4):422 e421–4.

14. Stevens T, van Wijngaarden E, Ackerman K, et al. Timing of delivery and survival rates for infants with prenatal diagnoses of congenital diaphragmatic hernia. Pediatrics 2009;123(2):494–502.

15. Congenital Diaphragmatic Hernia Study Group. Late-presenting congenital diaphragmatic hernia. J Pediatr Surg 2005;40(12):1839–43.

16. Colvin J, Bower C, Dickinson JE, et al. Outcomes of congenital diaphragmatic hernia: a population-based study in Western Australia. Pediatrics 2005;116(3):e356–63.

17. Hedrick HL, Crombleholme TM, Flake AW, et al. Right congenital diaphragmatic hernia: prenatal assessment and outcome. J Pediatr Surg 2004;39(3):319–23.

18. Scott DA. Genetics of congenital diaphragmatic hernia. Semin Pediatr Surg 2007;16(2):88–93.

19. Pober B. Genetic aspects of human congenital diaphragmatic hernia. Clin Genet 2008;74:1–15.

20. Bohn D. Congenital diaphragmatic hernia. Am J Respir Crit Care Med 2002;166:911–5.

21. Nobuhara K, Wilson J. Pathophysiology of congenital diaphragmatic hernia. Semin Pediatr Surg 1996;5(4):234–42.

22. Peralta C, Jani J, Cos T, et al. Left and right lung volumes in fetuses with diaphragmatic hernia. Ultrasound Obstet Gynecol 2006;27(5):551–4.

23. Adzick N, Harrison M, Glick P, et al. Diaphragmatic hernia in the fetus: prenatal diagnosis and outcome in 94 cases. J Pediatr Surg 1985;20(4):357–61.

24. Harrison M, Bressack M, Churg A, et al. Correction of congenital diaphragmatic hernia in utero. II. Simulated correction permits fetal lung growth with survival at birth. Surgery 1980;88(2):260–8.

25. Jesudason E, Connell M, Fernig D, et al. Early lung malformations in congenital diaphragmatic hernia. J Pediatr Surg 2000;35(1):124–7.

26. Kling DE, Schnitzer JJ. Vitamin A deficiency (VAD), teratogenic, and surgical models of congenital diaphragmatic hernia (CDH). Am J Med Genet C Semin Med Genet 2007;145C(2):139–57.

27. Willems P, Keersmaekers G, Dom K, et al. Fryns syndrome without diaphragmatic hernia? Am J Med Genet 1991;41(2):255–7.

28. Keijzer R, Liu J, Deimling J, et al. Dual-hit hypothesis explains pulmonary hypoplasia in the nitrofen model of congenital diaphragmatic hernia. Am J Pathol 2000;156(4):1299–306.

29. Shehata SM, Tibboel D, Sharma HS, et al. Impaired structural remodelling of pulmonary arteries in newborns with congenital diaphragmatic hernia: a histological study of 29 cases. J Pathol 1999;189(1):112–8.

30. Sakai H, Tamura M, Hosokawa Y, et al. Effect of surgical repair on respiratory mechanics in congenital diaphragmatic hernia. J Pediatr 1987;111(3):432–8.

31. Langham M, Krummel T, Bartlett R, et al. Mortality with extracorporeal membrane oxygenation following repair of congenital diaphragmatic hernia in 93 infants. J Pediatr Surg 1987;22:1150–4.

32. Lally K. Extracoporeal membrane oxygenation in patients with congenital diaphragmatic hernia. Semin Pediatr Surg 1996;5:249–55.

33. Langham M, Krummel T, Greenfield L, et al. Extracorporeal membrane oxygenation following repair of congenital diaphragmatic hernias. Ann Thorac Surg 1987;44:247–52.

34. Davis P, Firmin R, Manktelow B, et al. Long-term outcome following extracorporeal membrane oxygenation for congenital diaphragmatic hernia: the UK experience. J Pediatr 2004;144(3):309–15.

35. Wilson JM, Bower LK, Lund DP. Evolution of the technique of congenital diaphragmatic hernia repair on ECMO. J Pediatr Surg 1994;29(8):1109–12.

36. Lally K, Group CS. The use of ECMO for stabilization of infants with congenital diaphragmatic hernia. Paper presented at American Academy of Pediatrics, Surgical Section. Boston, October 19–23, 2002.

37. Lally KP, Paranka MS, Roden J, et al. Congenital diaphragmatic hernia. Stabilization and repair on ECMO. Ann Surg 1992;216(5):569–73.

38. Adolph V, Flageole H, Perreault T, et al. Repair of congenital diaphragmatic hernia after weaning from extracorporeal membrane oxygenation. J Pediatr Surg 1995;30(2):349–52.

39. Haricharan R, Barnhart D, Cheng H, et al. Identifying neonates at a very high risk for mortality among children with congenital diaphragmatic hernia managed with extracorporeal membrane oxygenation. J Pediatr Surg 2009;44(1):87–93.

40. Suda K, Bigras JL, Bohn D, et al. Echocardiographic predictors of outcome in newborns with congenital diaphragmatic hernia. Pediatrics 2000;105(5):1106–9.

41. Inhaled nitric oxide and hypoxic respiratory failure in infants with congenital diaphragmatic hernia. The Neonatal Inhaled Nitric Oxide Study Group. Pediatrics 1997;99(6):838–45.

42. Congenital Diaphragmatic Hernia Study Group. Does extracorporeal membrane oxygenation improve survival in neonates with congenital diaphragmatic hernia? J Pediatr Surg 1999;34(5):720–5.

43. Langer J, Filler R, Bohn D, et al. Timing of surgery for congenital diaphragmatic hernia: Is emergency operation necessary? J Pediatr Surg 1988;23(8):731–4.

44. Wung J, Sahni R, Moffitt S, et al. Congenital diaphragmatic hernia: survival treated with very delayed surgery, spontaneous respiration, and no chest tube. J Pediatr Surg 1995;30(3):406–9.

45. Joshi SB, Sudipta S, Chacko J, et al. Abdominal muscle flap repair for large defects of the diaphragm. Pediatr Surg Int 2005;21:677–80.

46. Mitchell I, Garcia N, Barber R, et al. Permacol: a potential biologic patch alternative in congenital diaphragmatic hernia repair. J Pediatr Surg 2008;43(12):2161–4.

47. Moss R, Chen C, Harrison M. Prosthetic patch durability in congenital diaphragmatic hernia: a long-term follow-up study. J Pediatr Surg 2001;36(1):152–4.

48. Grethel E, Cortes R, Wagner A, et al. Prosthetic patches for congenital diaphragmatic hernia repair: Surgisis vs Gore-Tex. J Pediatr Surg 2006;41(1):29–33.

49. Brant-Zawadzki PB, Fenton SJ, Nichol PF, et al. The split abdominal wall muscle flap repair for large congenital diaphragmatic hernias on extracorporeal membrane oxygenation. J Pediatr Surg 2007;42:1047–51.

50. Congenital Diaphragmatic Hernia Study Group. Defect size determines survival in infants with congenital diaphragmatic hernia. Pediatrics 2007;120(3):e651–7.

51. Taskin M, Zengin K, Unal E, et al. Laparoscopic repair of congenital diaphragmatic hernias. Surg Endosc 2002;16(5):869.

52. Holcomb GW 3rd, Ostlie DJ, Miller KA. Laparoscopic patch repair of diaphragmatic hernias with Surgisis. J Pediatr Surg 2005;40:E1–5.

53. Liem NT, Dung LA. Thoracoscopic repair for congenital diaphragmatic hernia: lessons from 45 cases. J Pediatr Surg 2006;41:1713–5.

54. Yang EY, Allmendinger N, Johnson SM, et al. Neonatal thoracoscopic repair of congenital diaphragmatic hernia: selection criteria for successful outcome. J Pediatr Surg 2005;40:1369–75.

55. Casaccia G, Crescenzi F, Palamides S, et al. Pleural effusion requiring drainage in congenital diaphragmatic hernia: incidence, aetiology and treatment. Pediatr Surg Int 2006;22(7):585–8.

56. Boloker J, Bateman D, Wung JT, et al. Congenital diaphragmatic hernia in 120 infants treated consecutively with permissive hypercapnea/spontaneous respiration/elective repair. J Pediatr Surg 2002;37(3):357–66.

57. Tiruvoipati R, Vinogradova Y, Faulkner G, et al. Predictors of outcome in patients with congenital diaphragmatic hernia requiring extracorporeal membrane oxygenation. J Pediatr Surg 2007;42:1345–50.

58. Khan AM, Lally KP. The role of extracorporeal membrane oxygenation in the management of infants with congenital diaphragmatic hernia. Semin Perinatol 2005;29:118–22.

59. Chiu P, Hedrick HL. Postnatal management and long-term outcome for survivors with congenital diaphragmatic hernia. Prenat Diagn 2008;28:592–603.

60. Austin MT, Lovvorn HN 3rd, Feurer ID, et al. Congenital diaphragmatic hernia repair on extracorporeal life support: a decade of lessons learned. Am Surg 2004;70(5):389–95 [discussion: 395].

61. Wilson JM, Bower LK, Fackler JC, et al. Aminocaproic acid decreases the incidence of intracranial hemorrhage and other hemorrhagic complications of ECMO. J Pediatr Surg 1993;28(4):536–40 [discussion: 540–1].

62. Downard CD, Betit P, Chang RW, et al. Impact of AMICAR on hemorrhagic complications of ECMO: a ten-year review. J Pediatr Surg 2003;38(8):1212–6.

63. Valls-i-Soler A, Alfonso L, Arnaiz A, et al. Pulmonary surfactant dysfunction in congenital diaphragmatic hernia: experimental and clinical findings. Biol Neonate 1996;69(5):318–26.

64. van Meurs KP, Congenital Diaphragmatic Hernia Study Group. Is surfactant therapy beneficial in the treatment of the term newborn infant with congenital diaphragmatic hernia? J Pediatr 2004;145:312–6.

65. Congenital Diaphragmatic Hernia Study Group. Surfactant does not improve survival rate in preterm infants with congenital diaphragmatic hernia. J Pediatr Surg 2004;39(6):829–33.

66. Colby CE, Congenital Diaphragmatic Hernia Study Group. Surfactant replacement therapy on ECMO does not improve outcome in neonates with congenital diaphragmatic hernia. J Pediatr Surg 2004;39(11):1632–7.

67. Cass DL. Fetal surgery for congenital diaphragmatic hernia: the North American experience. Semin Perinatol 2005;29:104–11.

68. Adzick N, Outwater K, Harrison M, et al. Correction of congenital diaphragmatic hernia in utero. IV. An early gestational fetal lamb model for pulmonary vascular morphometric analysis. J Pediatr Surg 1985;20(6):673–80.

69. Harrison M, Langer J, Adzick N, et al. Correction of congenital diaphragmatic hernia in utero. V. Initial clinical experience. J Pediatr Surg 1990;25(1):47–55.

70. Harrison MR, Adzick NS, Flake AW, et al. Correction of congenital diaphragmatic hernia in utero: VI. Hard-earned lessons. J Pediatr Surg 1993;28(10):1411–7.

71. Harrison M, Adzick N, Flake A, et al. Correction of congenital diaphragmatic hernia in utero. VIII: response of the hypoplastic lung to tracheal occlusion. J Pediatr Surg 1996;31(10):1339–48.

72. Kitano Y, Davies P, von Allmen D, et al. Fetal tracheal occlusion in the rat model of nitrofen-induced congenital diaphragmatic hernia. J Appl Phys 1999;87(2):769–75.

73. Skarsgard E, Meuli M, VanderWall K, et al. Fetal endoscopic tracheal occlusion ('Fetendo-PLUG') for congenital diaphragmatic hernia. J Pediatr Surg 1996;31(10):1335–8.

74. Deprest J, Gratacos E, Nicolaides K. Fetoscopic tracheal occlusion (FETO) for severe congenital diaphragmatic hernia: evolution of a technique and preliminary results. Ultrasound Obstet Gynecol 2004;24(2):121–6.

75. Harrison MRK, Roberta L, Hawgood SB, et al. A randomized trial of fetal endoscopic tracheal occlusion for severe fetal congenital diaphragmatic hernia. N Engl J Med 2003;349:1916–24.

76. Deprest J, Jani J, Gratacos E, et al. Fetal intervention for congenital diaphragmatic hernia: the European experience. Semin Perinatol 2005;29(2):94–109.

77. Wolfson MR, Shaffer TH. Pulmonary applications of perfluorochemical liquids: ventilation and beyond. Paediatr Respir Rev 2005;6(2):117–27.

78. Major D, Cadenas M, Cloutier R, et al. Combined gas ventilation and perfluorochemical tracheal instillation as an alternative treatment for lethal congenital diaphragmatic hernia in lambs. J Pediatr Surg 1995; 30(8):1178–82.

79. Pranikoff T, Gauger PG, Hirschl RB. Partial liquid ventilation in newborn patients with congenital diaphragmatic hernia. J Pediatr Surg 1996;31(5):613–8.

80. Nobuhara KK, Fauza DO, DiFiore JW, et al. Continuous intrapulmonary distension with perfluorocarbon accelerates neonatal (but not adult) lung growth. J Pediatr Surg 1998;33(2):292–8.

81. Fauza DO, Hirschl RB, Wilson JM. Continuous intrapulmonary distension with perfluorocarbon accelerates lung growth in infants with congenital diaphragmatic hernia: initial experience. J Pediatr Surg 2001;36(8):1237–40.

82. Hirschl RB, Philip WF, Glick L, et al. A prospective, randomized pilot trial of perfluorocarbon-induced lung growth in newborns with congenital diaphragmatic hernia. J Pediatr Surg 2003;38(3):283–9 [discussion: 283–9].

83. DeAnda AJ, Cahill J, Bernstein D, et al. Elective transplant pneumonectomy. J Pediatr Surg 1998; 33:655–6.

84. van Meurs K, Rhine W, Benitz W, et al. Lobar lung transplantation as a treatment for congenital diaphragmatic hernia. J Pediatr Surg 1994;29(12): 1557–60.

85. Azarow K, Messineo A, Pearl R, et al. Congenital diaphragmatic hernia—a tale of two cities: the Toronto experience. J Pediatr Surg 1997;32(3):395–400.

86. Wilson JM, Lund DP, Lillehei CW, et al. Congenital diaphragmatic hernia—a tale of two cities: the Boston experience. J Pediatr Surg 1997;32(3):401–5.

87. Bagolan P, Casaccia G, Crescenzi F, et al. Impact of a current treatment protocol on outcome of high-risk congenital diaphragmatic hernia. J Pediatr Surg 2004;39(3):313–8.

88. Midrio P, Gobbi D, Baldo V, et al. Right congenital diaphragmatic hernia: an 18-year experience. J Pediatr Surg 2007;42:517–21.

89. Muratore C, Utter S, Jaksic T, et al. Nutritional morbidity in survivors of congenital diaphragmatic hernia. J Pediatr Surg 2001;36(8):1171–6.

90. Chiu PP, Sauer C, Mihailovic A, et al. The price of success in the management of congenital diaphragmatic hernia: Is improved survival accompanied by an increase in long-term morbidity? J Pediatr Surg 2006;41(5):888–92.

91. Chen C, Jeruss S, Chapman JS, et al. Long-term functional impact of congenital diaphragmatic hernia repair on children. J Pediatr Surg 2007;42:657–65.

92. Diamond I, Mah K, Kim P, et al. Predicting the need for fundoplication at the time of congenital diaphragmatic hernia repair. J Pediatr Surg 2007;42(6):1066–70.

93. Su W, Berry M, Puligandla PS, et al. Predictors of gastroesophageal reflux in neonates with congenital diaphragmatic hernia. J Pediatr Surg 2007;42(10): 1639–43.

94. Chen C, Friedman S, Butler S, et al. Approaches to neurodevelopmental assessment in congenital diaphragmatic hernia survivors. J Pediatr Surg 2007; 42:1052–6.

95. Jaillard S, Pierrat V, Dubois A, et al. Outcome at 2 years of infants with congenital diaphragmatic hernia: a population-based study. Ann Thorac Surg 2003;75(1):250–6.

96. Cortes RA, Keller RL, Townsend T, et al. Survival of severe congenital diaphragmatic hernia has morbid consequences. J Pediatr Surg 2005;40(1):34–46.

Foramen of Morgagni Hernia: Presentation and Treatment

Ahmed Nasr, MD, MS, FRCSC[a], Annie Fecteau, MD, MHSc, FRCSC[b],*

KEYWORDS

• Morgagni • Hernia • Diaphragm • Retrosternal • Repair

Congenital diaphragmatic hernia (CDH) is a rare congenital anomaly characterized by a defect in diaphragm development with subsequent herniation of abdominal contents into the thorax. Two types are most prevalent, herniation anteriorly in the diaphragm (Morgagni hernia) and posterolateral (Bochdalek-type) hernias.

In 1769, Morgagni first described the rare anterior, retrosternal diaphragmatic defect that now bears his name. He noted this condition in the autopsy of an Italian stonecutter who died from gangrenous colon herniated through an opening beneath the sternocostal junction. There being no evidence of obstruction or trauma to the diaphragm, Morgagni concluded that "it had been thus from the original formation."[1] Because Napoleon's surgeon, Larrey, described a surgical approach to the pericardial sac through an anterior retrosternal diaphragmatic defect, these areas have been termed the Larrey spaces.

EMBRYOLOGY OF THE DIAPHRAGM

The diaphragm originates from an unpaired ventral portion (septum transversum), from paired dorsal lateral portions (pleuroperitoneal folds), and from an irregular medial dorsal portion (dorsal mesentery). The pericardial region is separated from the rest of the body by the septum transversum, formed during the third week of gestation. This part of the diaphragm grows dorsad from the ventral body wall and moves caudad with the other contributors to the diaphragm to reach the normal position of the diaphragm at about 8 weeks. The pleuroperitoneal folds arise on the lateral body walls, at the level where the cardinal veins swing around to enter the sinus venosus of the heart. These folds extend medially and somewhat caudad to join with the septum transversum and the dorsal mesentery to complete the development of the diaphragm at about the seventh week; the right pleuroperitoneal canal closes somewhat earlier than the left. Muscle fibers migrate from the third, fourth, and fifth cervical myotomes, carrying along their innervation, and grow between the two membranes to complete the structures of the diaphragm. A delay or variation in the described timetable may result in a variety of congenital hernias with or without a hernial sac, or may even result in a congenital eventration of a hemidiaphragm. Early return of the intestines to the abdomen before closure of the pleuroperitoneal membrane results in a hernia through this opening (a so-called foramen of Bochdalek hernia). Foramen of Morgagni hernias occur anteriorly, usually have a sac, and probably result from lack of ingrowth of the cervical myotomes.[2–5]

The foramen of Morgagni is a retrosternal space resulting from the failure of fusion of the fibrotendinous portion of the pars tendinalis arising from the costochondral arches with the fibrotendinous portion of the pars sternalis. This creates a defect between the sternal and costal origin of the diaphragm. This space is usually filled with fat and covered by pleura superiorly and peritoneum inferiorly. When present it offers a path through which abdominal viscera can herniate into the chest.

[a] Division of Pediatric Surgery, Hospital for Sick Children, 555 University Avenue, Toronto, Ontario, Canada M5G 1X8

[b] Division of Pediatric Surgery, University of Toronto, Hospital for Sick Children, 555 University Avenue, Toronto, Ontario, Canada M5G 1X8

* Corresponding author.

E-mail address: annie.fecteau@sickkids.ca (A. Fecteau).

Thorac Surg Clin 19 (2009) 463–468
doi:10.1016/j.thorsurg.2009.08.010
1547-4127/09/$ – see front matter © 2009 Elsevier Inc. All rights reserved.

INCIDENCE OF ASSOCIATED ANOMALIES

Morgagni hernia is the least common of the congenital diaphragmatic defects occurring with a varied frequency of 1% to 5.1% in a large series. Clinically evident hernias through the foramen of Morgagni are uncommon at any age. Despite their congenital etiology, they are detected less often in children than in adults.[1,6–8] Harrington[8] listed only seven foramen of Morgagni hernias (1.5%) in a series of 430 patients who were operated on for diaphragmatic hernia. Out of a total of 750 patients with diaphragmatic hernias of all kinds found over 32 years, Comer and Clagett[9] reported 50 patients (7%) with foramen of Morgagni hernias. Overall, the incidence of Morgagni hernia among all diaphragmatic defects in adults and children is 3% to 4%. Morgagni hernias are far more common on the right despite protection from the liver. About 90% of the hernias occur on the right, 8% are bilateral, and only 2% are limited to the left.[10] One hypothesis for this disparity is that the more extensive pericardial attachments on the left provide additional support for that side of the diaphragm. The defect itself usually has a greater transverse dimension than the anteroposterior dimension. Foramen of Morgagni hernias are detected more often in women than in men and more often in obese people than in those of average or below-average weight.[5]

When Morgagni hernia presents in infancy, it usually is accompanied by one or more anomalies. In one study, 13 of 17 patients had significant congenital defects, including cardiac defects such as dextrocardia, ventricular septal defect, anomalous pulmonary venous return, trisomy 21, and large omphaloceles. Liver, colon, and small bowel often are found in the hernia in infants, in contrast to the adult presentation, in which omental fat is often the only structure in the hernia and there are no associated congenital anomalies.[6,11]

SYMPTOMS

Berardi[12] reported that about one third of patients are asymptomatic in a literature review of 132 adult and pediatric cases. The most common contents of the hernia sac are colon, small bowels, liver, omentum, and stomach. Patients with symptoms most frequently describe chronic gastrointestinal complaints, such as crampy pain or constipation from partial intermittent colonic obstruction. On the other hand, symptoms due to intermittent gastric volvulus or small bowel obstruction are less frequent. Patients often complain only of vague epigastric or substernal fullness or a dull,

right-subcostal discomfort. Complete obstruction, incarceration, or strangulation with necrosis of a hollow viscus contained in a foramen of Morgagni hernia is rare and is associated with an acute or subacute presentation. In the aforementioned series, 12 patients had complete bowel obstruction, and 1 had gangrenous intestine.[5,9,12]

Cardiorespiratory symptoms such as dyspnea and palpitations are less common overall than gastrointestinal complaints. Although children are more often asymptomatic than adolescents and adults, they have about an equal incidence of respiratory and gastrointestinal symptoms.

As with other hernias, conditions that produce prolonged or sudden, severe, increased intra-abdominal pressure can precipitate the onset of, or exacerbate, existing symptoms due to a foramen of Morgagni hernia. Exercise and athletic activity were reported by Valases and Sills[13] as a cause the occurrence of symptoms. Ellyson and Parks[14] reported that trauma could initiate symptoms. Lin and Maginot[15] described a patient who became symptomatic during pregnancy.

The vast majority of the cases of Morgagni hernia are detected in asymptomatic children and adults. Vague epigastric discomfort may be the only symptom in many cases. Rarely, the hernia presents in neonates and infants, in whom symptoms such as respiratory distress and cyanosis could be present. Like the Bochdalek hernias at a similar age, other manifestations include cough, choking episodes, vomiting following feeds, constipation, diarrhea, failure to thrive, postprandial fullness, and respiratory infections. Some cases may be discovered incidentally by visualizing the air-fluid levels or solid masses in the retrosternal region or on the right side of the chest radiograph. Many cases may remain undetected and present only later in life. This may be because, though the defect is present from birth, presence of a sac resists herniation through the defect. Rupture of the sac by trauma or raised intra-abdominal pressure allows herniation and development of symptoms. Alternatively, viscera may be herniated at an early stage, but the patient remains asymptomatic until bowel complications occur. It has been noted that congenital diaphragmatic hernia discovered before 2 years of age are more likely to be symptomatic.[5,8,16,17]

When a child with Down syndrome presents to the physician with respiratory distress, congenital heart disease, lower respiratory tract infection, gastroesophageal reflux and lung anomalies are commonly considered depending upon the clinical settings. Unawareness on the part of the treating physician about occurrence of Morgagni hernia in Down syndrome may be responsible for delayed detection.

A literature search revealed several cases of Down syndrome that had associated Morgagni hernia. The age of presentation varied from neonatal to 12 years. The mode of presentation varied from asymptomatic detection to the presentation with respiratory distress. Identical twins with Down syndrome with identical heart disease and Morgagni hernia have been reported.[7,18,19]

Although these cases represent only a small percentage of patients with Morgagni hernia, this suggests that there may be a genetic component to Morgagni hernia. This significant association between the hernia of Morgagni and trisomy 21 may reflect defective dorsoventral migration of rhabdomyoblasts from the paraxial myotomes, caused by increased cellular adhesiveness in trisomy 21.[18,19]

This association has clinical implications. In addition to screening for congenital heart disease, hypothyroidism, and refractive errors, the screening procedure for Morgagni hernia may also be undertaken—especially in the cases of Down syndrome with respiratory manifestations. In cases of Morgagni hernia, the physician would have to be careful to look for cases of mosaic Down that may be missed clinically.

Postnatally, other than respiratory distress, clinical examination is usually unrewarding in detection of Morgagni hernia. Although a chest radiograph may raise suspicions about the presence of Morgagni hernia, the diagnosis should be confirmed by barium studies, ultrasonography, radionuclide scan, or CT scan. Incarceration and strangulation are the complications of an unrepaired hernia and occur in 10% of cases.

DIAGNOSIS

The diagnosis of a foramen of Morgagni hernia is made by radiography, either prompted by symptoms or performed for unrelated reasons. In very small hernias, "the sign of the cane" was described by Lanuza.[20] It is a curvilinear accumulation of fat continuous with the properitoneal fat line of the anterior abdominal wall. This sign suggests that a small anterior cardiophrenic mass may be a foramen of Morgagni hernia. However, the standard chest radiograph may show an obvious right, left, or bilateral pericardiophrenic abnormalities that are solid or contain air, depending on the herniated organ. The usual finding is a rounded opacity at the right cardiophrenic angle. The lateral chest film localizes this density to the anterior retrosternal space. The

opacification is generally due to omentum rising through the hernia defect. An air-fluid level may be seen on chest film when the transverse colon, small bowel, or stomach herniate through the defect. In adults, pericardial cyst, prominent fat pad, loculated pneumothorax, bronchial carcinoma in the cardiophrenic region, and atypical mediastinal tumor may mimic the radiographic features of herniation through the foramen of Morgagni.[20–23]

Contrast studies of the colon or upper gastrointestinal tract can confirm the diagnosis in patients with visceral herniation. CT scan is diagnostic in cases with or without visceral herniation because it demonstrates the presence of fat, a hollow viscus, or both, without the need for gastrointestinal contrast. The usual CT finding is a retrosternal mass of fat density representing herniated omentum or a combination of omentum and an air-containing viscus. An MRI can provide similar information but is usually not required. Although radiographs after induced pneumoperitoneum have been used to outline the hernia sac for definitive diagnosis, this approach is rarely needed and is of historic interest only.[21,22]

An air-filled viscus in the mediastinum on plain chest radiograph is the single most common scenario. Given the lack of symptoms, these patients are generally older than those with Bochdalek hernias. The hernia most often contains liver, but transverse colon, stomach, and small intestine are possible. Incarcerated hollow viscera usually account for any related symptoms.

CT is used to identify the location of the hernia and to determine whether and how much stomach, bowel, and mesentery has herniated into the chest. Occasionally a portion of bowel may lie within the hernial sac. In the latter instance, it may be possible to make the diagnosis on routine roentgenographic study of the chest, but a CT or sonographic study usually is required to confirm the diagnosis. If omentum is herniated, the fat can be identified. Other studies include barium enema, which may show upward angulation of the midtransverse colon when the hernial sac contains omentum. The pyloric end of the stomach and proximal duodenum may also be displaced upward toward the diaphragm.[5,23,24]

Rarely, in infants and young children the liver may herniate through the foramen of Morgagni into the thorax. This is usually accompanied by partial obstruction of the inferior vena cava. Inferior vena cavography demonstrates the kinking and partial obstruction of the inferior vena cava.

The differential diagnosis of a mass in the anterial cardiophrenic angle on imaging includes a pleuropericardial cyst, pleural mesothelioma, hiatal hernia, large anterior mediastinal masses, Bochdalek hernia, and pericardial fat pad. Patients on a high dose of steroids frequently have an enlarged pericardial fat pad, which can be easily confused with a foramen of Morgagni hernia.

The anomaly can be diagnosed antenatally, albeit uncommonly.

MANAGEMENT

Lung hypoplasia is not commonly encountered in cases of Morgagni hernia as compared with the Bochdalek type. However, if this is encountered in the neonate, an ICU with an intensivist who has the experience in management of these cases is needed.

Management options for these patients encompass a number of different modalities, and there is no consensus on a single best approach.

Surgical Repair

Surgery provides definitive management for patients with Morgagni hernia. However, because the low prevalence of Morgagni hernia, it is impossible to compare operative and nonoperative management. Hence, the true benefit of surgery is unknown.

It is easy to justify surgery for symptomatic patients, so the real quandary lies with the management of asymptomatic patients. Those who advocate surgery for asymptomatic patients believe that the hernias may enlarge over time and there is always a low, but definite, risk of progression to incarceration and strangulation. Thus, a safe, elective operation can become a potentially high-risk procedure. Whereas Hunter[25] described successful nonoperative management of a Morgagni hernia, there are several examples of patients who have failed this management strategy. One of these patients was followed for 18 years by Jemerin[26] before requiring surgery.[8,26-29] In some asymptomatic cases, however, it is reasonable to follow the patient without repair. This group includes people with only herniated omentum who have comorbidities that increase the risk for operation.

Several surgical approaches have been used to repair Morgagni hernias. The abdominal approach allows for easier reduction of the hernia contents, evaluation of the contralateral diaphragm for additional defects, and concomitant evaluation and repair of intraabdominal pathology. An abdominal approach repair is generally performed through an upper midline, subcostal, or paramedian incision. A midline approach allows easy access to both sides in the event that bilateral hernias are encountered. Adhesions are taken down, and the contents of the hernia are reduced into the peritoneal cavity. The margins of the hernia sac are identified, and the sac is generally resected. As in all types of hernia surgery, a tension-free closure is required to prevent recurrence. For small defects that can be closed primarily, repair of the muscular defect is performed with heavy, interrupted, nonabsorbable mattress sutures. Prosthetic patches are used to close larger defects. In many patients, it is not necessary to enter the chest or to drain the pleural space.[17,25,30-33] Boyd and Wooldridge[33] described a patient who underwent thoracotomy, then experienced an intestinal obstruction 2 years later through the contralateral defect that was not visualized. In addition, in the event that the abdomen cannot accommodate the hernia contents, use of the abdominal approach allows the surgeon to repair the defect and leave a ventral hernia, which can be addressed later. A higher complication rate and a longer hospital stay after laparotomy may be explained by the fact that most emergency operations are performed through this approach.

The primary advantage of the thoracic approach is that it provides easier dissection of the hernia sac off the mediastinal and pleural structures. Despite the more widespread use of laparoscopy, thoracotomy continues to be the most widely used surgical approach for Morgagni hernias reported in the literature.[17,31-33]

Boyd and Wooldridge[33] reported a thoracic approach in 9 of 10 patients of his series; whereas Comer and Clagett[9] strongly recommended the abdominal approach if the diagnosis was made preoperatively. Coexisting pathology and experience of the operator may be a factor in deciding which approach to use.

Occasionally, a foramen of Morgagni hernia is encountered during a thoracotomy performed for an undiagnosed mediastinal mass or other indication. Once identified, the sac is opened and explored, and the contents are reduced into the peritoneal cavity. Primary or prosthetic patch repair of the defect can often be performed in a manner similar to the transabdominal technique. In some cases, adequate repair requires passing the sutures around a rib anteriorly or through the sternal periosteum.

Successful repair during pregnancy also has been reported. Kurzel and colleagues[34] recommend elective repair if Morgagni hernia is discovered in the first or second trimesters. If it is discovered in the third trimester, a mature fetus should be ensured before simultaneous cesarean section and hernia repair are performed.

Management of the hernia sac is controversial.[32] Ramachandran and Arora[35] reported complete resolution of an unexcised sac by CT scan 1 month postoperatively. However, during the same time interval, the patient studied by Contini and colleagues[36] still had a small residual cyst as seen by CT scan. Some investigators think the hernia sac should not be resected, while others prefer a more selective approach and recommend removing the sac only when it is small, without intrathoracic adhesions, and when the chance of injuring thoracic structures is low. Still, some feel resection of the sac is safe and adhere more strictly to classic surgical principles.

The role of minimally invasive surgery is evolving. The technique for laparoscopic repair of Morgagni hernia has been well described. The patient is placed in reverse Trendelenburg position and three to five ports are placed with an orientation similar to that for a laparoscopic Nissen fundoplication or other upper abdominal surgery. It is important not to place trocars too close to the costal margin.[17] To avoid tension, Thoman and colleagues[32] recommend using prosthetic mesh to cover defects larger than 20 to 30 cm^2. Others recommend using mesh repairs in all cases except those involving neonates. Several different types of materials have been used: polypropylene, expanded polytetrafluoroethylene (dual mesh; Gore Medical, Flagstaff, AZ, USA), Composix (C. R. Bard, Inc, Murray Hill, NJ, USA), and Parietex (Parietex Composite; Sofradim, Trevoux, France), to name a few.[37–41]

Mesh fixation can be performed with surgical tacks or various laparoscopic suturing techniques. If polypropylene mesh is used to repair the defect, some surgeons do not cover the mesh because they think the liver and omentum provide ample protection for the bowel. This concept may not apply to left-sided hernias.[35,42] However, tissue coverage of the mesh can be achieved with omentum, peritoneal flap, or falciform ligament or ligamentum teres. Additionally, repair has been accomplished laparoscopically without pneumoperitoneum by using an abdominal wall-lifting device.[43–45]

Experience is increasing with minimally invasive approaches to the treatment of foramen of Morgagni hernias. The results of surgical repair of foramen of Morgagni hernias are excellent. Operative mortality and morbidity are low, especially for elective repair. There were five deaths (3.8%), involving one child and four adults, in the series of 132 patients reviewed by Berardi and colleagues.[12] Of paramount importance is that all five deaths occurred in patients with strangulated bowel. Although there are no reliable data on recurrence rates, individual reports of recurrences are rare. Follow-up is limited, but the results of laparoscopic repair appear to be excellent so far.

SUMMARY

Morgagni hernias are rare and most often asymptomatic. However, there is always a concern about strangulated bowel. Diagnosis is usually by chest radiograph or CT scan. The surgical approach may be either transabdominal or thoracic. There are increasing reports about the role of minimally invasive approach. The recurrence is low with an excellent prognosis.

REFERENCES

1. Ronald B. Ponn. Foramen of Morgagni hernia chapter 52. General Thoracic Surgery. 6th edition. Philadelphia: Lippincott Williams and Wilkins; 2004.
2. Thomas W. Shields. Embryology and anatomy of the diaphragm. chapter 48. General Thoracic Surgery. 6th edition. Philadelphia: Lippincott Williams and Wilkins; 2004.
3. Anson BJ. Atlas of human anatomy. Philadelphia: WB Saunders; 1950.
4. Anson BJ, McVay C. Surgical anatomy. 5th edition. Philadelphia: WB Saunders; 1971.
5. Patten B. Human embryology. 3rd edition. New York: McGraw-Hill; 1968. p. 406.
6. Pokorny WJ, McGill CW, Harberg FJ. Morgagni hernias during infancy: presentation and associated anomalies. J Pediatr Surg 1984;19:394–7.
7. Synder WH, Greaney EM. Congenital diaphragmatic hernias; 77 consecutive cases. Surgery 1965;57: 567–88.
8. Harrington SW. Various types of diaphragmatic hernia treated surgically. Surg Gynecol Obstet 1948;86:735.
9. Comer TP, Clagett OT. Surgical treatment of hernia of the foramen of Morgagni. J Thorac Cardiovasc Surg 1966;52:461.
10. Stolar CJH, Dillon PW. Congenital diaphragmatic hernia and eventration. In: O'Neill JA, Rowe MI, Grosfeld JL, et al, editors. Paediatric surgery. 5th edition. St. Louis (MO): C.V. Mosby; 1998. p. 819–37.
11. Berman L, Stringer D, Ein SH, et al. The late-presenting paediatric Morgagni hernia: a benign condition. J Pediatr Surg 1989;24:970–2.
12. Berardi RS, Tenquist J, Sauter D, et al. An update on the surgical aspects of Morgagni hernia. Surg Rounds 1997;370–6.
13. Valases C, Sills C. Case report: anterior diaphragmatic hernia (hernia of Morgagni). N J Med 1988; 85:603.
14. Ellyson JH, Parks SN. Hernia of Morgagni in trauma patients. J Trauma 1986;26:569.

15. Lin JC, Maginot AE. Postpartum incarcerated Morgagni's hernia: an unusual presentation of Morgagni's hernia. Surg Rounds 1999;70–2.

16. Naunheim KS. Adult presentation of unusual diaphragmatic hernias. Chest Surg Clin N Am 1998;8:359.

17. Horton JD, Hofmann LJ, Hetz SP. Presentation and management of Morgagni hernia in adults: a review of 298 cases. Surg Endosc 2008;22(6):1413–20.

18. Parmar RC, Tullu MS, Bavdekar SB, et al. Morgagni hernia with Down syndrome: a rare association. Case report and review of literature. J Postgrad Med 2001;47.

19. Harris GJ, Soper RT, Kimura KK. Foramen of Morgagni hernia in identical twins: is this an inheritable defect? J Pediatr Surg 1993;28:177–8.

20. Lanuza A. The sign of the cane: a new radiological sign for the diagnosis of small Morgagni hernias. Radiology 1981;101:293.

21. Hussong RL, Landreneau RJ, Cole FH. Diagnosis and repair of a Morgagni hernia with video-assisted thoracic surgery. Ann Thorac Surg 1997;63:1474.

22. Loong TP, Kocher HM. Clinical presentation and operative repair of hernia of Morgagni. Postgrad Med J 2005;81:41–4.

23. Fernandez-Cebrian JM, De Oteyza JP. Laparoscopic repair of hernia of foramen of Morgagni. J Laparoendosc Surg 1996;6:61.

24. Kuster GGR, Kline LE, Garzo G. Diaphragmatic hernia through the foramen of Morgagni: laparoscopic repair. J Laparoendosc Surg 1992;2:93.

25. Hunter WR. Herniation through the foramen of Morgagni. Br J Surg 1959;47:22–7.

26. Jemerin EE. Diaphragmatic hernia through the foramen of Morgagni. J Mt Sinai Hosp N Y 1963; 30:415–26.

27. Dalvi AN, Rege SA, Ravikiran CS, et al. Laparoscopic repair of Morgagni hernia in adult. Indian J Gastroenterol 2001;20:70.

28. Meredith K, Allen J, Richardson JD, et al. Foramen of Morgagni hernia: surgical consideration. J Ky Med Assoc 2000;98:286–8.

29. White DC, McMahon R, Wright T, et al. Laparoscopic repair of a Morgagni hernia presenting with syncope in an 85-year-old woman: case report and update of the literature. J Laparoendosc Adv Surg Tech A 2002;12:161–5.

30. Minneci PC, Deans KJ, Kim P, et al. Foramen of Morgagni hernia: changes in diagnosis and treatment. Ann Thorac Surg 2004;77:1956–9.

31. Slaetis P. Herniation through the foramen of Morgagni: clinical observations in 17 operatively treated cases. Ann Chir Gynaecol Fenn 1963;52:477–86.

32. Thoman DS, Hui T, Phillips EH. Laparoscopic diaphragmatic hernia repair. Surg Endosc 2002;16:1345–9.

33. Boyd DP, Wooldridge BF. Diaphragmatic hernia through the foramen of Morgagni. Surg Gynecol Obstet 1957;104:727–32.

34. Kurzel RB, Naunheim KS, Schwartz RA. Repair of symptomatic diaphragmatic hernia during pregnancy. Obstet Gynecol 1988;71:869–71.

35. Ramachandran CS, Arora V. Laparoscopic transabdominal repair of hernia of Morgagni-Larrey. Surg Laparosc Endosc Percutan Tech 1999;9:358–61.

36. Contini S, Dalla Valle R, Bonati L, et al. Laparoscopic repair of a Morgagni hernia: report of a case and review of the literature. J Laparoendosc Adv Surg Tech 1999;9:93.

37. Mouroux J, Venissac N, Alifano M, et al. Morgagni hernia and thoracic deformities. Thorac Cardiovasc Surg 2003;51:44–5.

38. Settembre A, Cuccurullo D, Pisaniello D, et al. Laparoscopic repair of congenital diaphragmatic hernia with prosthesis: a case report. Hernia 2003;7:52–4.

39. Marin-Blazquez AA, Candel MF, Parra PA, et al. Morgagni hernia: repair with a mesh using laparoscopic surgery. Hernia 2004;8:70–2.

40. Yavuz N, Yigitbasi R, Sunamak O, et al. Laparoscopic repair of Morgagni hernia. Surg Laparosc Endosc Percutan Tech 2006;16:173–6.

41. Bortul M, Calligaris L, Gheller P. Laparoscopic repair of a Morgagni-Larrey hernia. J Laparoendosc Adv Surg Tech 1998;8:309–13.

42. Del Castillo D, Sanchez J, Hernandez M, et al. Morgagni's hernia resolved by laparoscopic surgery. J Laparoendosc Adv Surg Tech 1998;8:105–8.

43. Nguyen T, Eubanks PJ, Nguyen D, et al. The laparoscopic approach for repair of Morgagni hernia. JSLS 1998;2:85–8.

44. Rau HG, Schardey HM, Lange V. Laparoscopic repair of a Morgagni hernia. Surg Endosc 1994;8:1439–42.

45. Orita M, Okino M, Yamashita K, et al. Laparoscopic repair of a diaphragmatic hernia through the foramen of Morgagni. Surg Endosc 1997;11:668–706.

Congenital Diaphragmatic Hernia in the Adult

Lana Schumacher, MD, Sebastien Gilbert, MD*

KEYWORDS

- Congenital diaphragmatic hernia • Adult
- Bochdalek • Morgagni • Laparoscopic

Congenital diaphragmatic herniae (CDH) are rare, occurring in 1 of 3000 live births.[1] The true prevalence in the adult population remains unknown. Autopsy studies estimated the prevalence in adults to be 1:7000 to 1:2000, whereas reviews of computed tomographic (CT) scans estimated the prevalence to be as high as 6%.[2,3]

CDH occur when there is a developmental defect of the diaphragm's muscular components. The diaphragmatic defect may allow displacement of abdominal viscera into the thorax during fetal development. This usually leads to impaired pulmonary embryogenesis and symptomatic presentation early in life. However, a small subset of patients may not develop symptoms until adulthood.

The most common type of CDH is a posterolateral defect in the diaphragm, named Bochdalek hernia after it was first described by Victor Alexander Bochdalek in 1848 among neonates presenting with signs and symptoms of respiratory distress. The incidence of posterolateral diaphragmatic herniae has been estimated to be 1:12,500 to 1:2200 live births. The diagnosis of Bochdalek hernia in adults is extremely rare and less than 200 patients have been reported. One study reported an incidence of 0.17% based on 13,138 abdominal CT scan reports reviewed in 1 year. Adults most commonly present with complaints of abdominal pain rather than respiratory symptoms.[4] In neonates, 85% of these defects are left-sided. In adults, right-sided Bochdalek hernia occurs more frequently, although the left side still predominates. The liver may prevent early herniation of the abdominal viscera through right-sided defects and hence delay the onset of symptoms until later in life, which may account for the apparent increased frequency of right-sided Bochdalek hernias in adults.[2,5,6]

A second type of CDH, Morgagni hernia, is less common than Bochdalek hernia, and is often diagnosed incidentally in adults.[7] In the eighteenth century, Morgagni first described a substernal herniation of abdominal contents into the thoracic cavity based on observations made during autopsy examinations.[4] Morgagni herniae are anterior and usually right-sided. The anterior portion of the left hemidiaphragm is protected from herniation by the overlying pericardial sac, which may explain the right-sided predominance. They may occur bilaterally and, unlike Bochdalek herniae, they are usually lined by a peritoneal sac. The authors know of no large retrospective or prospective studies providing data on the prevalence or incidence of Morgagni hernia in adults. Neurologic and congenital heart anomalies may coexist in 40% to 50% of patients.[8] Morgagni herniae may also be associated with chromosomal abnormalities, such as Turner syndrome and trisomy 13, 18, and 21.[9]

EMBRYOLOGY

The diaphragm develops from 4 embryologic sources as outlined in a previous article. Bochdalek herniae result from the improper fusion of the septum transversum and pleuroperitoneal folds.[10] Morgagni herniae are thought to result from failure

Division of Thoracic Surgery, Heart, Lung, and Esophageal Surgery Institute, UPMC Presbyterian, Suite C-800, 200 Lothrop Street, Pittsburgh, PA 15213, USA
* Corresponding author.
E-mail address: gilbsx@upmc.edu (S. Gilbert).

Thorac Surg Clin 19 (2009) 469–472
doi:10.1016/j.thorsurg.2009.08.004

of fusion of the anterior costal elements with the sternal components.

CLINICAL PRESENTATION

Conditions associated with increased intraabdominal pressure, such as pregnancy and obesity, may lead to progressive enlargement of the diaphragmatic defect and herniation of abdominal contents into the thorax.[11] The more common presenting symptoms include shortness of breath, food intolerance with postprandial emesis, gastroesophageal reflux, intermittent nausea, vomiting, abdominal cramping, distension, and nonspecific abdominal pain. The most common contents of diaphragmatic hernia are omentum (92%), colon (58%), and stomach (25%).[12] One-fourth to half of all CDH in adults are diagnosed incidentally.[12,13] Clinical characteristics of CDH in adults are summarized in **Table 1**. The presentation of CDH in adults differs from neonates. In neonates, Bochdalek herniae are characteristically left-sided and have a male predominance. In adults, a higher proportion of Bochdalek herniae present on the right side of the diaphragm and they occur more commonly in women. Morgagni herniae are often associated with predisposing factors that lead to increased intraabdominal pressure (obesity, pregnancy, constipation).

Complications, such as volvulus, incarceration, strangulation, hemorrhage, or visceral perforation, have all been described.[6,14] These cases require immediate surgical attention and signs of incarceration and strangulation are considered surgical emergencies. Other atypical presentations have been reported and include tension pneumothorax due to a colo-pleural fistula from an incarcerated Bochdalek hernia, pancreatitis, and splenic rupture.[10,15,16] There are also rare reports of incarceration during pregnancy.[17] Therefore, antepartum repair of asymptomatic CDH has been recommended. Corticosteroids should be given to the mother before surgery to promote fetal lung maturation, if the fetus gestational age is between 24 and 34 weeks.[18]

RADIOLOGIC FINDINGS

Herniated bowel loops with air fluid levels in the hemithorax and elevation of the diaphragm are pathognomonic signs. Chest radiographs, CT scans, and barium enema studies are useful diagnostic modalities. CT is considered the preferred diagnostic modality; however, a normal scan does not exclude the diagnosis.[19] For left-sided defects, the reported sensitivity of CT scanning is 78% and the specificity is 100%.[20] For right-sided defects, the sensitivity is 50% and specificity is 100%.[20] **Figs. 1** and **2** provide examples of CT scan findings for each type of CDH.

SURGICAL REPAIR

All diaphragmatic herniae should be repaired at the time of diagnosis, given the risk of intestinal obstruction and strangulation. Traditionally, CDH have been repaired via laparotomy or thoracotomy. Minimally invasive approaches may also provide excellent exposure for repair and may have additional benefits, such as decreased pain, shorter hospitalization, and improved cosmesis.[21,22]

Minimally invasive repair of CDH can be performed either thoracoscopically or laparoscopically. The thoracoscopic approach is preferred by some for its excellent visualization and ease of reduction of hernia contents. The thoracoscopic approach also provides good exposure to the hernia sac and allows safe dissection of potential pericardial and pleural adhesions.[23] Patients considered for thoracoscopic repair should undergo a gastrointestinal contrast study to exclude the presence of malrotation. The presence of malrotation is a contraindication to the thoracoscopic approach, because it is difficult to

Table 1
Patient characteristics and laterality of Bochdalek and Morgagni hernia in adults[5,13]

	Bochdalek	Morgagni
Mean age (years)	66	53
Women (%)	77	62
Predisposing factors (%)[a]	–	41
Right-sided (%)	68	91
Left-sided (%)	18	5
Bilateral (%)	14	4

[a] Predisposing factors: pregnancy, trauma, obesity, chronic constipation, and chronic cough.

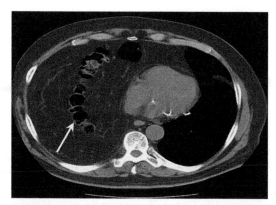

Fig. 1. Right-sided Bochdalek hernia containing omentum and transverse colon (*arrow*) in an 80-year-old man who had dyspnea for many years. Patient had an open repair with mesh.

assess orientation of reduced abdominal contents.[19,22] The main advantage of the laparoscopic approach is that the hernia contents are visualized more easily once reduced in the abdomen. Therefore, if there is a high degree of suspicion of intestinal incarceration and ischemia, it may be more appropriate to use a minimally invasive or open transabdominal approach.[21,24] Primary closure with interrupted, nonabsorbable suture is the preferred method of repair, when the diaphragmatic edges can be apposed without undue tension. The use of mesh has been recommended when the size of the diaphragmatic defect exceeds 20 to 30 cm^2.[12,25,26]

Recurrence rates are low for all approaches (laparotomy, thoracotomy, laparoscopy, and thoracoscopy) and outcomes have been excellent. A retrospective review of 298 cases of Morgagni hernia repair reported 1 recurrence over a mean

follow-up between 12 and 85 months.[13] There were no recurrences in a series of 12 patients during a 6-month to 10-year follow-up after repair of a Morgagni hernia.[12] Furthermore, studies comparing the minimally invasive approach with open repair show no difference in recurrences with either approach. A study evaluating open repair with thoracotomy and laparotomy yielded 1 recurrence out of 207 patients. The same investigators also reviewed the recurrences following either thoracoscopy or laparoscopy; the review showed no recurrences in 48 patients. Follow-up time was 58 to 109 months in the open repair group versus 12 to 15 months in the minimally invasive group.[13] Given the small size of published surgical series and the lack of comparative data, it is difficult to determine if the open or minimally invasive approaches, or primary repair, or repair with mesh reinforcement provides superior long-term results.[13,25,27]

At the University of Pittsburgh Medical Center, 10 adult patients have undergone elective surgical repair of a CDH over the past 11 years. The mean age at presentation was 71 years (range, 61–80 years) and 80% presented with symptoms of either abdominal discomfort or dyspnea, but no patient had an incarcerated or strangulated hernia. All were initially approached using thoracoscopy (n = 3) or laparoscopy (n = 7), and 3 (30%) were ultimately converted to an open repair. Four patients had a Bochdalek hernia (3 right-sided and 1 left-sided). Of these, the right-sided defects were approached with video-assisted thoracoscopy, but 2 of the 3 eventually converted to open procedures. The reasons for conversion to thoracotomy were (1) pleural adhesions from previous thoracotomy for a lung resection and (2) extremely large defect. The one left-sided Bochdalek hernia was repaired laparoscopically. Six patients had a Morgagni hernia, 2 left-sided and 4 right-sided defects. Most of the Morgagni defects (83.3%; 5 of 6) were successfully repaired using laparoscopy. Mesh reinforcement was used in 5 patients and primary repair was used in 1 patient with a small defect. There was 1 conversion to laparotomy for repair of an intestinal injury. There were no recurrences at a median follow-up of 18 months (range, 2–115 months).

SUMMARY

Bochdalek hernia is a rare surgical condition primarily diagnosed in infants. Morgagni hernia is more commonly identified in adults. A subset of patients with a Bochdalek hernia, especially those with a right-sided defect, may also be diagnosed during adulthood. Both adult forms of CDH may

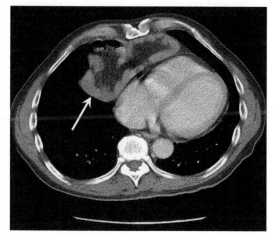

Fig. 2. Morgagni hernia in a 72-year-old man containing normal caliber ileum (*arrow*). This hernia was diagnosed incidentally.

be discovered incidentally or diagnosed as part of the investigation of nonspecific gastrointestinal or respiratory symptoms. It is recommended that all adult CDH patients undergo surgical repair to prevent incarceration and strangulation of abdominal viscera. Currently, many reports have demonstrated the safety and efficacy of using open or minimally invasive repair techniques, with or without mesh reinforcement. Regardless of the approach selected, surgical repair has been associated with low morbidity and mortality and excellent long-term outcomes with low rate of recurrence.

REFERENCES

1. Langham MR Jr, Kays DW, Ledbetter DJ, et al. Congenital diaphragmatic hernia. Epidemiology and outcome. Clin Perinatol 1996;23(4):671–88.
2. Gale ME. Bochdalek hernia: prevalence and CT characteristics. Radiology 1985;156(2):449–52.
3. Salacin S, Alper B, Cekin N, et al. Bochdalek hernia in adulthood: a review and an autopsy case report. J Forensic Sci 1994;39(4):1112–6.
4. Morgagni GB. Founders of modern medicine: Giovanni Battista Morgagni. (1682–1771). Med Library Hist J 1903;1(4):270–7.
5. Mullins ME, Stein J, Saini SS, et al. Prevalence of incidental Bochdalek's hernia in a large adult population. AJR Am J Roentgenol 2001;177(2):363–6.
6. Bujanda L, Larrucea I, Ramos F, et al. Bochdalek's hernia in adults. J Clin Gastroenterol 2001;32(2):155–7.
7. Rogers FB, Rebuck JA. Case report: Morgagni hernia. Hernia 2006;10(1):90–2.
8. Tibboel D, Gaag AV. Etiologic and genetic factors in congenital diaphragmatic hernia. Clin Perinatol 1996;23(4):689–99.
9. Naunheim KS. Adult presentation of unusual diaphragmatic hernias. Chest Surg Clin N Am 1998; 8(2):359–69.
10. Raichoudhury RC, Patnaik SC, Sahoo M, et al. Foramen of Bochdalek hernia in adults. Chest 1973;64(2):259–62.
11. Thomas TV. Subcostosternal diaphragmatic hernia. J Thorac Cardiovasc Surg 1972;63(2):279–83.
12. Minneci PC, Deans KJ, Kim P, et al. Foramen of Morgagni hernia: changes in diagnosis and treatment. Ann Thorac Surg 2004;77(6):1956–9.
13. Horton JD, Hofmann LJ, Hetz SP. Presentation and management of Morgagni hernias in adults: a review of 298 cases. Surg Endosc 2008;22(6):1413–20.
14. Al-Emadi M, Helmy I, Nada MA, et al. Laparoscopic repair of Bochdalek hernia in an adult. Surg Laparosc Endosc Percutan Tech 1999;9(6):423–5.
15. Harrington DK, Curran FT, Morgan I, et al. Congenital Bochdalek hernia presenting with acute pancreatitis in an adult. J Thorac Cardiovasc Surg 2008; 135(6):1396–7.
16. Robb BW, Reed MF. Congenital diaphragmatic hernia presenting as splenic rupture in an adult. Ann Thorac Surg 2006;81(3):e9–10.
17. Gimovsky ML, Schifrin BS. Incarcerated foramen of Bochdalek hernia during pregnancy. A case report. J Reprod Med 1983;28(2):156–8.
18. Genc MR, Clancy TE, Ferzoco SJ, et al. Maternal congenital diaphragmatic hernia complicating pregnancy. Obstet Gynecol 2003;102(5 Pt 2): 1194–6.
19. Silen ML, Canvasser DA, Kurkchubasche AG, et al. Video-assisted thoracic surgical repair of a foramen of Bochdalek hernia. Ann Thorac Surg 1995;60(2): 448–50.
20. Killeen KL, Mirvis SE, Shanmuganathan K. Helical CT of diaphragmatic rupture caused by blunt trauma. AJR Am J Roentgenol 1999;173(6): 1611–6.
21. Palanivelu C, Rangarajan M, Senthilkumar R, et al. Laparoscopic surgery for giant adult Bochdalek diaphragmatic hernia: combined suturing and polypropylene mesh repair. J Coll Physicians Surg Pak 2007;17(8):502–4.
22. Yamaguchi M, Kuwano H, Hashizume M, et al. Thoracoscopic treatment of Bochdalek hernia in the adult: report of a case. Ann Thorac Cardiovasc Surg 2002;8(2):106–8.
23. Kilic D, Nadir A, Doner E, et al. Transthoracic approach in surgical management of Morgagni hernia. Eur J Cardiothorac Surg 2001;20(5):1016–9.
24. Craigie RJ, Mullassery D, Kenny SE. Laparoscopic repair of late presenting congenital diaphragmatic hernia. Hernia 2007;11(1):79–82.
25. Palanivelu C, Rangarajan M, Rajapandian S, et al. Laparoscopic repair of adult diaphragmatic hernias and eventration with primary sutured closure and prosthetic reinforcement: a retrospective study. Surg Endosc 2009;23(5):978–85.
26. Kitano Y, Lally KP, Lally PA. Late-presenting congenital diaphragmatic hernia. J Pediatr Surg 2005; 40(12):1839–43.
27. Nguyen TL, Le AD. Thoracoscopic repair for congenital diaphragmatic hernia: lessons from 45 cases. J Pediatr Surg 2006;41(10):1713–5.

Paraesophageal Hernia: Clinical Presentation, Evaluation, and Management Controversies

Colin Schieman, MD, FRCSC, Sean C. Grondin, MD, MPH, FRCSC*

KEYWORDS
- Hiatal hernia • Paraesophageal hernia
- Repair • Management • Giant paraesophageal hernia

There are many types of diaphragmatic hernias and the terminology used to classify them is often confusing. The common feature of all is that some portion of the stomach has been displaced into the thorax. Anatomically, there are hernias through the diaphragmatic esophageal hiatus and those distinct from the hiatus. The latter are more correctly called "parahiatal diaphragmatic" hernias, the classic examples being congenital hernias through the diaphragmatic muscle proper, such as a Bochdalek or Morgagni hernia. This article addresses hernias through the esophageal hiatus. When describing hiatal hernias, the authors favor the traditional classification, which defines the hiatal hernia according to the position of the gastroesophageal junction (GEJ) and the extent of herniated stomach.[1]

Type I hiatal hernia is a sliding hernia that occurs with migration of the GEJ into the posterior mediastinum through the hiatus because of laxity of the phrenoesophageal ligament (**Fig. 1**). This type accounts for more than 95% of hiatal hernias.[2,3] Most small type I sliding hernias are asymptomatic. When they enlarge, the predominant symptom is gastroesophageal reflux.[4]

Type II is a true paraesophageal hernia (PEH), which occurs when the fundus herniates through the hiatus alongside a normally positioned GEJ by a defect in the phrenoesophageal membrane (**Fig. 2**). This is the least common type of hiatal hernia.[5]

Type III is a combination of types I and II hernias with cranially displaced GEJ and stomach through the hiatus (**Fig. 3**). As the hiatal hernia enlarges and more stomach herniates, volvulus of the intrathoracic stomach may develop because of tethering of the lesser curve of the stomach by the gastrohepatic omentum and left gastric vessels.

Type IV is a hernia characterized by displacement of the stomach with other organs, such as the colon, spleen, and small bowel into the chest.

Although this classification is commonly used in the literature and accurately describes the anatomic spectrum of hiatal hernias, from a practical perspective these patients are divided into those with sliding hiatal hernias (type I) and those with PEHs (any one of types II, III, or IV). The literature on PEHs rarely specifies the type of hiatal hernia with authors typically grouping types II, III, and IV together. Distinguishing between these types of hernias is important, however, because type II usually does not require a gastroplasty, whereas types III or IV hernias may require an esophageal lengthening procedure.[6] For the purposes of this article the focus is primarily on the management of type II to IV hernias, referred to collectively as "paraesophageal" hernias.

Division of Thoracic Surgery, Foothills Hospital, University of Calgary, 1403 29th Street NW, Calgary, Alberta T2N 2T9, Canada
* Corresponding author.
E-mail address: sean.grondin@albertahealthservices.ca (S.C. Grondin).

Thorac Surg Clin 19 (2009) 473–484
doi:10.1016/j.thorsurg.2009.08.006

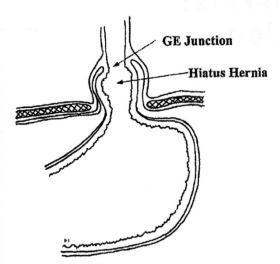

Fig. 1. Type I sliding hernia. (*From* Ilves R. Hiatus hernia: the condition. Chest Surg Clin N Am 1998;8:404; with permission.)

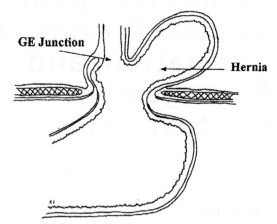

Fig. 3. Type III paraesophageal hernia. Larger hernia with GEJ above the diaphragm. (*From* Ilves R. Hiatus hernia: the condition. Chest Surg Clin N Am 1998;8:404; with permission.)

CLINICAL PRESENTATION

Although the exact figure is unknown, it is estimated that approximately 50% of patients with PEH are asymptomatic.[5] Confounding the issue is the presence of symptoms that are often nonspecific, minor in severity, and incorrectly ascribed to the "aging process" in this generally elderly patient population. A thorough history often uncovers symptoms related to PEH that were not previously reported on less detailed questioning. When present, symptoms and complications of PEH are reflective of the mechanical alterations caused by the hernia. Broadly, symptoms are either caused by obstruction or by gastroesophageal reflux resulting from a dysfunctional lower esophageal sphincter (LES).

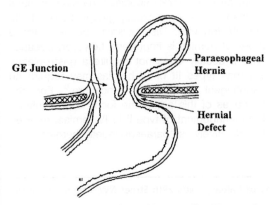

Fig. 2. Type II paraesophageal hernia. The GEJ remains below the diaphragm. (*From* Ilves R. Hiatus hernia: the condition. Chest Surg Clin N Am 1998;8:404; with permission.)

Mechanical obstruction of either the distal esophagus or stomach can result in dysphagia, epigastric pain, vomiting, postprandial fullness, early satiety, or dyspnea. Dysphagia and postprandial discomfort are the most commonly reported symptoms, occurring in more than 50% of symptomatic patients.[7–9] These symptoms may be minor and episodic, or become severe and unremitting. Occasionally, patients may present with severe epigastric pain caused by incarceration and gastric obstruction. If obstruction persists the stomach distends and ischemia, perforation, and septic shock may ensue. In 1904, Borchardt[10] described a triad of symptoms seen in patients with acute obstruction from PEH that included chest pain, retching with inability to vomit, and inability to pass a nasogastric tube. This rare acute presentation represents a surgical emergency.

Dysfunctional LES resulting from displacement of the stomach into the chest may cause symptoms related to gastroesophageal reflux disease (GERD). Although not as common as symptoms caused by mechanical obstruction, GERD symptoms, such as heartburn, chronic cough, regurgitation, and aspiration, may be reported on careful history.

Important signs associated with PEH are recurrent pneumonia from aspiration and iron deficiency anemia from chronic blood loss. This bleeding may be secondary to esophagitis caused by GERD but more frequently is caused by erosions or ulcerations of the mucosa at an area of gastric folding,[5,11,12] called Cameron lesions or ulcers.[13] This anemia resolves in greater than 90% of patients following repair of the hernia.[14,15]

EVALUATION

Evaluation of a patient with a known or suspected PEH depends on the acuity of the presentation and surgeon preference. The goals of the diagnostic evaluation are to establish or confirm the diagnosis of PEH, define the anatomy of the hernia, rule out associated pathologies, and determine the presence or absence of GERD.

Plain chest radiograph often identifies a PEH by revealing a retrocardiac air-fluid level within the intrathoracic stomach. In the acutely unwell patient radiographs may reveal evidence of gastric compromise and perforation manifested as pneumomediastinum or pneumoperitoneum. CT of the chest and abdomen may also provide additional information on the type and location of the hernia.

The most important test in establishing a diagnosis of PEH is the upper gastrointestinal (UGI) series. Key information obtained from this contrast study is the anatomic location of the esophagus and stomach and, more specifically, the position of the GEJ. In some cases, the UGI series reveals complete obstruction caused by gastric volvulus. This radiographic finding indicates a patient requiring urgent surgical intervention.[16]

Endoscopy should be performed on all patients being evaluated for PEH. Esophagoscopy rules out associated pathologies and establishes the diagnosis of PEH while defining the location of the GEJ and the size and type of hernia. In type I hernias, the GEJ and gastric pouch extend above the impression made by the diaphragmatic crura, whereas in a type II hernia there is a separate orifice containing protruded stomach adjacent to a normally located GEJ. A type III hernia may be suspected on endoscopy when a large gastric pouch is seen above the diaphragm with the GEJ entering midway along the side of the pouch. Accurately defining the anatomy of a large hernia may be difficult, however, because of the inability to pass the scope through the stomach and into the antrum.

The use of manometry in the evaluation of PEH is controversial. Proponents of manometry believe that this test allows the LES to be precisely localized resulting in a more accurate classification of the type of hernia.[5,17] Manometry may also be helpful in assessing the patient for esophageal shortening by measuring the intersphincteric distance between the upper esophageal sphincters and LES.[7] Further, manometry can evaluate the peristaltic function of the esophageal body, which may rule out an undiagnosed motility disorder and the function of the LES, which may assist the surgeon in tailoring an antireflux procedure to a specific patient.[12,18,19] Others argue that manometry adds little to the preoperative work-up with other investigations, such as endoscopy and UGI series, able to confirm the diagnosis and classify the type of hernia. Manometry may be technically difficult to perform, with some authors noting an inability to complete the testing in more than 50% of patients with PEH.[18,19] Finally, preoperative manometric findings do not influence most surgeons' decision to perform an esophageal lengthening procedure or fundoplication when repairing a PEH.

Similarly, ambulatory pH testing in patients with PEH is not usually required[12,18] because most patients have reflux on pH testing.[20,21] Most surgeons also routinely perform a fundoplication as part of the PEH repair; pH testing does not alter the planned operation.[22]

MANAGEMENT

In the acute setting, most surgeons agree that urgent surgical intervention is indicated. In the chronic setting there is debate about indications for surgery and the best operative approach. Controversy also exists regarding the need for an esophageal lengthening procedure, fundoplication, fixation of the stomach with gastropexy or gastrostomy, and the need for prosthetic reinforcement of the hiatal closure.

Indications for Surgery

Traditionally, elective surgical repair has been recommended for all patients with PEH considered to be medically operable.[17,23,24] Part of the rationale for this recommendation is based on the tendency of PEH to enlarge with time making surgery more difficult and the increasing age of the patient, which may increase the risk of complications. Some surgeons also think that patients with PEH have a high rate of developing lethal complications.[25] In the classic report by Skinner and Belsey[25] 29% (6 of 21) of patients with documented PEH who were observed with minimal symptoms died from complications of strangulation, perforation, or bleeding. In a recent retrospective study by Allen and coworkers[26] 23 of 147 patients were followed after refusing surgery and none of them developed a life-threatening complication of their PEH. Only 4 of these 23 patients ultimately developed progressive symptoms requiring operation. This suggests that a selective approach to surgery is appropriate, with surgery reserved for patients who are symptomatic.[18,27,28] Some surgeons believe that emergency repair of PEH is associated with a high mortality rate. In 1973, Hill[29] reported a series of patients with acute gastric volvulus associated with PEH that had an operative mortality rate of 56%. This high mortality rate provided further impetus to repair all PEH regardless of symptoms. Several recent reports, however, including a pooled analysis by Stylopoulos and coworkers,[28] demonstrate a much lower mortality rate (5%–17%) for emergency surgery.[30–35] In light of this information, it seems reasonable that asymptomatic or minimally symptomatic patients do not necessarily require surgery and that a more selective approach should be used.[36–38] There remains little debate, however, that all symptomatic patients who are a good surgical risk should be repaired.[38,39]

Approach to Surgery

The three approaches for repair of PEH are (1) transthoracic, (2) transabdominal, and (3) laparoscopic. Regardless of the approach, the tenets for a successful repair of PEH are tension-free reduction of hernia contents into the subdiaphragmatic position, removal of the hernia sac, and closure of the hiatal defect.[40] Most surgeons also agree that performing an antireflux procedure is an important element of a successful PEH repair. The role of fixation of the stomach below the diaphragm with gastropexy or gastrostomy is debated.

Traditionally, PEH repair was through a thoracotomy or laparotomy. Proponents of the thoracic approach emphasized the ease of dissection of the hernia sac and its contents and the enhanced ability to fully mobilize the esophagus to reduce tension and minimize the need for a lengthening procedure. If a lengthening procedure is required, it is generally easier with the thoracic approach. The thoracic repair has the disadvantages of being associated with increased pain and pulmonary complications postoperatively, the need for tube thoracostomy, increased hospital stay and cost, and the potential for volvulus after reduction of the stomach into the abdomen.[40–42]

Advocates of the abdominal approach argue that it permits complete mobilization of the stomach with improved reduction of the volvulus and recreation of the normal anatomy. This approach also allows other abdominal procedures, such as gastropexy or gastrostomy, to be performed. Mobilization of the distal esophagus can be challenging, however, making gastroplasty for esophageal shortening more difficult to perform.[42]

There are no randomized studies comparing open abdominal with thoracic approaches in the repair of PEH. **Table 1** lists the outcomes of several studies of PEH repair using either technique.[7,27,33,43–49] Comparing these series is difficult because of variable clinical and radiographic follow-up and different and inconsistent outcome measures. Low and Unger[48] report the highest rate of recurrence (18%) with most recurrences being asymptomatic. This result likely represents a true estimate of anatomic recurrence based on the thorough follow-up investigations performed by the authors. Despite these differences, these studies indicate that both transthoracic and transabdominal approaches have good outcomes with low postoperative mortality rates and acceptable rates of recurrence.

The first report of laparoscopic repair of PEH was published in 1992.[50] Today there is far more published literature on minimally invasive repair of PEH than on all the open series combined. Advocates of the laparoscopic approach claim that it has decreased postoperative morbidity and affords superior visualization of the hiatus and mediastinum, which allows better distal esophageal mobilization.[22,42] Arguments against this approach include the advanced laparoscopic skills required to perform the surgery, the lack of long-term follow-up, and a higher recurrence rate of PEH.[22,40] There are no randomized control trials comparing laparoscopic with open PEH repair to support these claims.

At the authors' institution the short-term outcomes of primary laparoscopic and open PEH repairs were evaluated in 93 patients.[51] The primary outcome measures included intraoperative parameters, such as operative time, and postoperative variables, such as hospital stay and complications. Secondary outcomes included mortality rates, recurrence rates, and patient satisfaction. It was concluded that the laparoscopic approach was associated with a significantly longer operative time (3.1 hours) compared with the open procedure (2.5 hours). The overall hospital stay was shorter in the laparoscopic group (5 days), however, compared with the open repair group (10 days) and was associated with fewer postoperative complications. Although the follow-up was short (average 17 months), the patient satisfaction scores and recurrence rates (9%) were similar in both groups.

Table 2 lists the outcomes of several studies using the laparoscopic approach for repair of PEH.[52–59] Advocates of the minimally invasive approach cite series that demonstrate decreased length of stay, lower postoperative complication rates, and lower mortality rates than the open repair. In a review of 32 different case series, Draaisma and coworkers[24] reported a lower perioperative complication rate and a shorter mean length of stay for the laparoscopic versus the open group (3 versus 10 days). Rathore and

Table 1
Outcomes of selected series of open thoracic and abdominal repair of PEH

	References	Year	N	% Lengthening Gastroplasty	% Good or Excellent Results	% Anatomic Recurrence	Follow-up (Months)
Transthoracic repair	Allen et al[26]	1993	124	68	93	NR	42 (median)
	Maziak et al[7]	1998	94	80	94	2	72 (median)
	Altorki et al[44]	1998	47	0	91	6	45 (median)
	Patel et al[45]	2004	240	96	85	8	42 (median)
Transabdominal repair	Williamson et al[46]	1993	119	1	84	11	61 (median)
	Myers et al[47]	1995	37	0	92	0.3	67 (median)
	Low and Unger[48]	2005	72	0	NR	18	30 (mean)
Mixed series	Martin et al[49]	1997	51	NR	86	4	27 (mean)
	Geha et al[33]	2000	100	2	98	0	NR

Abbreviation: NR, not reported.

Adapted from Parekh KR, Iannettoni MD. Lengthening gastroplasty for managing giant paraesophageal hernia. In: Ferguson MK, editor. Difficult decisions in thoracic surgery: an evidence-based approach. 1st edition. London: Springer-Verlag; 2007. p. 318–22; with permission.

Table 2
Outcomes of selected series of laparoscopic repair of PEH

Author	Year	N	% Lengthening Gastroplasty	% Anatomic Recurrence	Follow-up (Months)
Trus et al[52]	1997	76	8	11	15 (median)
Wiechmann et al[53]	2001	60	0	7	40 (mean)
Mattar et al[54]	2002	136	5	43	18 (median)
Pierre et al[55]	2002	203	56	2	37 (mean)
Jobe et al[56]	2002	52	0	32	37 (mean)
Diaz et al[57]	2003	116	5	32	30 (mean)
Andujar et al[58]	2004	166	0	5	15 (mean)
Boushey et al[59]	2008	58	0	9	6 (mean)

Adapted from Parekh KR, Iannettoni MD. Lengthening gastroplasty for managing giant paraesophageal hernia. In: Ferguson MK, editor. Difficult decisions in thoracic surgery: an evidence-based approach. 1st edition. London: Springer-Verlag; 2007. p. 318–22; with permission.

coworkers[60] published a meta-analysis of non-randomized series on laparoscopic PEH repair. Inclusion was restricted to those series with greater than 25 patients and follow-up beyond 6 months. In 965 patients the overall recurrence rate was 10.2%. Among those patients formally evaluated with a contrast esophagogram postoperatively 25.5% had recurrence. Lower recurrence rates were seen in those who underwent an esophageal lengthening procedure with a Collis-Nissen gastroplasty versus those who did not (0% vs 12%). Despite both the widespread adoption of laparoscopic techniques for various procedures and the impressive published results, laparoscopic repair of PEH has not been universally adopted. In a recent international online survey of members of the Cardiothoracic Surgery Network only 48% stated they repair PEH laparoscopically, whereas 35% perform thoracotomy and 17% perform laparotomy.[61]

The debate surrounding the best surgical approach for repairing PEH continues with several studies reporting that each approach can be performed safely with acceptable outcomes.

Esophageal Shortening

The true incidence of esophageal shortening in PEH is unknown and remains a major point of controversy. Despite having been described for over 50 years,[62] questions remain as to the existence and the management of a shortened esophagus. Those who believe that shortening does not exist argue that in most patients the esophagus appears shortened because the stomach is pushing it up into the chest. Correction of the anatomic arrangement avoids the need for a lengthening procedure.[63] A more commonly held view is that although short esophagus is uncommon, it remains an important cause of recurrence following PEH repair.[18,64] Inadequate esophageal length limits the ability to reduce the GEJ into its normal abdominal position without tension, which predisposes to wrap herniation and anatomic recurrence.[64]

The most important risk factor for esophageal shortening is the presence of periesophageal inflammation resulting from long-standing GERD.[64] It is thought that GERD leads to chronic irritation followed by healing and subsequent fibrosis.[65] Studies of patients diagnosed with GERD demonstrate a wide range of incidence of short esophagus (0%–60%).[66–68] Other risk factors that may predispose a patient to develop esophageal shortening include Barrett esophagus, scleroderma, and Crohn disease.[65,68]

Identifying patients preoperatively with shortened esophagus is problematic.[69,70] There is no test that can be performed that accurately identifies the presence and degree of esophageal shortening. Several techniques have been described using endoscopic or radiologic measurements of length and manometric measurements.[70–73] Unfortunately, none of these are completely reliable at predicting a shortened esophagus intraoperatively.[70,74,75] The most reliable method of determining esophageal shortening is intraoperative assessment (eg, GEJ >2.5 cm below the hiatus).[64,75]

When a diagnosis of short esophagus is made a lengthening procedure is necessary. This may be accomplished by further intrathoracic dissection and mobilization of the esophagus or by gastroplasty. In 1957, Collis[76] described this procedure without fundoplication. Subsequently, fundoplication was added to prevent reflux and is referred to as Collis-Nissen.[77] Although a Collis-Nissen is most easily done by thoracotomy, it can be performed through any approach.[78,79] There is general agreement that a lengthening gastroplasty reduces the rate of recurrent herniation following repair of PEH when esophageal shortening is observed.[6,43]

Esophageal shortening is less commonly identified in patients undergoing laparoscopic repair of PEH.[22] This observation may be related to difficulty in accurately identifying the GEJ because of inadequate removal of the fat pad, elevation of the diaphragm from insufflation of carbon dioxide, or improved distal esophageal mobilization.[6] Some surgeons may also be reluctant to perform a gastroplasty using laparoscopic techniques because of technical challenges. Long-term follow-up of patients undergoing laparoscopic repair of PEH is necessary to determine if decreased use of gastroplasty in the laparoscopic approach results in higher recurrence rates.

Antireflux Procedure

Although limited data confirm the need for fundoplication, most surgeons perform an antireflux procedure when repairing a PEH[24] because the fundoplication helps to anchor the stomach in the abdomen and because of the need to recreate a barrier to reflux. The extensive dissection necessary for full mobilization of the hernia sac and esophagus completely disrupts the hiatal mechanism and may render the GEJ incompetent resulting in postoperative reflux. An incidence of postoperative reflux as high as 65% in patients who did not receive a fundoplication has been reported.[37,63,80] These results have been disputed and a few argue that significant postoperative reflux is much less common in patients without fundoplication and, if present, can be managed with medical therapy.[46] Some authors believe that avoiding a fundoplication decreases the risk of postoperative dysphagia and operative complications, and shortens the operative time for patients who are often elderly with significant medical comorbidities.[81] These authors suggest that fundoplication should be performed selectively in patients diagnosed with GERD on preoperative evaluation.

Fixation of the Stomach with Gastropexy or Gastrostomy

In many patients, reherniation occurs because of positive intra-abdominal pressure and negative intrathoracic pressure creating a cephalad force that favors migration of the stomach into the thorax. By anchoring the stomach below the diaphragm by gastropexy or gastrostomy, it is hoped that this migration is avoided.[63] Surgeons who argue for gastropexy note that it is fast and simple to perform; however, a high rate of recurrence has been reported using this technique.[22,82,83] Those who favor gastrostomy argue that it provides a solid anchoring point to prevent recurrence and decreases the risk of intra-abdominal gastric volvulus.[22] Gastrostomy also effectively decompresses the stomach and eliminates the need for a nasogastric tube postoperatively. Those surgeons who oppose fixation of the stomach report that reherniation is not prevented because the stomach is pliable and merely stretches in response to the cephalad force.[22] No prospective randomized study has been reported that proves that either of these two techniques reduces the rate of recurrence.

Mesh Reinforcement of the Crural Repair

PEH repair is often complicated by excessive tension of the hiatal closure, attenuated crura with poor quality tissue, and unrecognized esophageal shortening. These factors predispose the crural repair to disruption and lead to reherniation. To improve the strength of the crural repair, surgeons have used prosthetic mesh. This approach is supported by the successful use of mesh for the repair of inguinal and incisional hernias. In these patients, the mesh causes secondary in-growth and fibrosis and significantly reduces the incidence of hernia recurrence.[84–86]

Data supporting the use of prosthetics for crural reinforcement during PEH repair are limited because most studies are small observational case series using different techniques of repair and different prosthetic materials.[87] Three techniques for mesh placement have been described with each intended to provide mechanical support to the hiatal closure: (1) primary closure of the crura followed by prosthetic onlay,[88] (2) the "keyhole" technique whereby a slit and hole are cut into the mesh and it is placed around the esophagus onto the crura,[89] and (3) the "tension free" repair whereby the hiatal defect is left open and mesh is used to bridge the gap between the crura.[90]

Prosthetic insertion may cause complications including erosion into the esophagus, adhesions, fibrotic strictures, and dysphagia.[91–94] Prosthetic erosion is rare but catastrophic and may require esophagectomy as definitive management.[88,91–94] To address these concerns, biologic mesh, such as porcine small intestinal submucosa and

Table 3
Outcomes of selected series of laparoscopic repair of PEH with mesh prosthesis

	References	Year	N	% Recurrence	Prosthetic Material	Placement of Mesh	Follow-up (Months)
Nonrandomized trials	Basso et al[90]	2000	65 NM 70 M	14 0	PP	Tension free	23
	Hui et al[97]	2001	12 NM 12 M	0 8	PTFE	Onlay	37
	Champion and Rock[98]	2003	52 M	2	PP	Onlay	25
	Keidar and Szold[99]	2003	23 NM 10 M	17 10	Composite	Keyhole	58
Randomized trials	Frantzides et al[89]	2002	36 NM 36 M	23 0	PTFE	Keyhole	40
	Granderath et al[88]	2005	50 NM 50 M	26 8	PP	Onlay	12
	Oelschlager et al[100]	2006	57 NM 51 SM	24 9	Porcine SIS	Onlay	6

Abbreviations: M, mesh; NM, no mesh; PP, polypropylene; PTFE, polytetrafluoroethylene; SIS, small intestinal submucosa; SM, synthetic mesh.
Adapted from Davis SS Jr. Current controversies in paraesophageal hernia repair. Surg Clin North Am 2008;88:959–78; with permission.

acellular human dermis, have been investigated.[22,40] Theoretically, these materials are safer because they act as infection-resistant temporary scaffolding that allows for native tissue in-growth without the degree of scarring created by synthetic mesh.[95,96]

Despite the drawbacks listed previously, there is increasing evidence[90,97–99] including two prospective randomized controlled trials[88,89] suggesting that mesh reinforcement of crural closure decreases the risk of reherniation (**Table 3**). Oelschlager and coworkers[100] demonstrated similar results using bioprosthetic mesh with no mesh-related complications reported. Long-term follow-up is required to ensure that erosion into the esophagus does not occur with newer materials.

SUMMARY

Practically, hiatal hernias are divided into sliding hiatal hernias (type I) and PEH (types II, III, or IV). Patients with PEH are usually symptomatic with GERD or obstructive symptoms, such as dysphagia. Rarely, patients present with acute symptoms of hernia incarceration, such as severe epigastric pain and retching. A thorough evaluation includes a complete history and physical examination, chest radiograph, UGI series, esophagogastroscopy, and manometry. These investigations define the patient's anatomy, rule out other disease processes, and confirm the diagnosis. Operable symptomatic patients with PEH should be repaired. The underlying surgical principles for successful repair include reduction of hernia contents, removal of the hernia sac, closure of the hiatal defect, and an antireflux procedure. Debate remains whether a transthoracic, transabdominal, or laparoscopic approach is best with good surgical outcomes being reported with all three techniques. Placement of mesh to buttress the hiatal closure is reported to reduce hernia recurrence. Long-term follow-up is required to determine whether the laparoscopic approach with mesh hiatoplasty becomes the procedure of choice.

REFERENCES

1. Ilves R. Hiatus hernia: the condition. Chest Surg Clin N Am 1998;8(2):401–9.
2. Kahrilas PJ. Hiatus hernia causes reflux: fact or fiction? Gullet 1993;3(Suppl):21.
3. Peridikis G, Hinder RA. Paraesophageal hiatal hernia. In: Nyhus LM, Condon RE, editors. Hernia. Philadelphia: JB Lippincott; 1995. p. 544–54.
4. Mattioli S, D'Ovidio F, Di Simone MP, et al. Clinical and surgical relevance of the progressive phases of intrathoracic migration of the gastroesophageal junction in gastroesophageal reflux disease. J Thorac Cardiovasc Surg 1998;116(2):267–75.
5. Maish MS, Demeester SR. Paraesophageal hiatal hernia. In: Cameron J, editor. Current surgical therapy. 8th edition. Philadelphia: Elsevier Mosby; 2004. p. 38–42.
6. Darling G, Deschamps C. Technical controversies in fundoplication surgery. Thorac Surg Clin 2005; 15(3):437–44.
7. Maziak DE, Todd TR, Pearson FG. Massive hiatus hernia: evaluation and surgical management. J Thorac Cardiovasc Surg 1998;115(1):53–60.
8. Wo JM, Branum GD, Hunter JG, et al. Clinical features of type III (mixed) paraesophageal hernia. Am J Gastroenterol 1996;91(5):914–6.
9. Velanovich V, Karmy-Jones R. Surgical management of paraesophageal hernias: outcome and quality of life analysis. Dig Surg 2001;18(6):432–7.
10. Borchardt M. Zur pathologie und therapie des magenvolvulus [Pathology and therapy of gastric volvulus]. Arch Klin Chir 1904;74:243–60 [in German].
11. Peters JH, Demeester TR. Esophagus and diaphragmatic hernia. In: Brunicardi FC, Andersen DK, et al, editors. Schwartz's principles of surgery. 8th edition. New York: McGraw-Hill; 2005. p. 835–931.
12. Oelschlager BK, Eubanks TR, Pellegrini CA. Hiatal hernia and gastroesophageal reflux disease. In: Townsend CM, Beauchamp RD, Evers BM, et al, editors. Sabiston textbook of surgery. 18th edition. Philadelphia: WB Saunders; 2004. p. 1151–66.
13. Weston AP. Hiatal hernia with Cameron ulcers and erosions. Gastrointest Endosc Clin N Am 1996; 6(4):671–9.
14. Pauwelyn KA, Verhamme M. Large hiatal hernia and iron deficiency anaemia: clinico-endoscopical findings. Acta Clin Belg 2005;60(4):166–72.
15. Hayden JD, Jamieson GG. Effect on iron deficiency anemia of laparoscopic repair of large paraesophageal hernias. Dis Esophagus 2005;18(5): 329–31.
16. Bawahab M, Mitchell P, Church N, et al. Management of acute paraesophageal hernia. Surg Endosc 2009;23(2):255–9.
17. Naunheim KS, Limpert P. Paraesophageal hiatal hernia. In: Shields TW, LoCicero J, Ponn RB, et al, editors. General thoracic surgery. 6th edition. Philadelphia: Lippincott Williams & Wilkins; 2004. p. 2190–9.
18. Maziak DE, Pearson FG. Massive (paraesophageal) hiatal hernia. In: Patterson GA, Cooper JD, Deslauriers J, et al, editors. Pearson's thoracic and esophageal surgery. 3rd edition. Philadelphia: Churchill Livingstone; 2008. p. 233–8.

19. Swanstrom LL, Jobe BA, Kinzie LR, et al. Esophageal motility and outcomes following laparoscopic paraesophageal hernia repair and fundoplication. Am J Surg 1999;177(5):359–63.

20. Fuller CB, Hagen JA, DeMeester TR, et al. The role of fundoplication in the treatment of type II paraesophageal hernia. J Thorac Cardiovasc Surg 1996;111(3):655–61.

21. Walther B, Demeester TR, Lafontaine E, et al. Effect of paraesophageal hernia on sphincter function and its implication on surgical therapy. Am J Surg 1984;147(1):111–6.

22. Wolf PS, Oelschlager BK. Laparoscopic paraesophageal hernia repair. Adv Surg 2007;41:199–210.

23. Kahrilas PJ. Hiatus Hernia. UpToDate Online 17.1; Available at: www.uptodate.com/online/content/topic.do?topicKey=eso_dis/4849&selectedTitle=1~49&source=search_result. Updated December 15, 2008. Accessed March 30, 2009.

24. Draaisma WA, Gooszen HG, Tournoij E, et al. Controversies in paraesophageal hernia repair: a review of literature. Surg Endosc 2005;19(10):1300–8.

25. Skinner DB, Belsey RH. Surgical management of esophageal reflux and hiatus hernia: long-term results with 1,030 patients. J Thorac Cardiovasc Surg 1967;53(1):33–54.

26. Allen MS, Trastek VF, Deschamps C, et al. Intrathoracic stomach: presentation and results of operation. J Thorac Cardiovasc Surg 1993;105(2):253–8.

27. Floch NR. Paraesophageal hernias: current concepts. J Clin Gastroenterol 1999;29(1):6–7.

28. Stylopoulos N, Gazelle GS, Rattner DW. Paraesophageal hernias: operation or observation? Ann Surg 2002;236(4):492–500.

29. Hill LD. Incarcerated paraesophageal hernia: a surgical emergency. Am J Surg 1973;126(2):286–91.

30. Carter R, Brewer LA, Hinshaw DB. Acute gastric volvulus: a study of 25 cases. Am J Surg 1980;140(1):99–106.

31. Haas O, Rat P, Christophe M, et al. Surgical results of intrathoracic gastric volvulus complicating hiatal hernia. Br J Surg 1990;77(12):1379–81.

32. Menguy R. Surgical management of large paraesophageal hernia with complete intrathoracic stomach. World J Surg 1988;12(3):415–22.

33. Geha AS, Massad MG, Snow NJ, et al. A 32-year experience in 100 patients with giant paraesophageal hernia: the case for abdominal approach and selective antireflux repair. Surgery 2000;128(4):623–30.

34. Ozdemir IA, Burke WA, Ikins PM. Paraesophageal hernia: a life-threatening disease. Ann Thorac Surg 1973;16(6):547–54.

35. Beardsley JM, Thompson WR. Acutely obstructed hiatal hernia. Ann Surg 1964;159:49–62.

36. Horgan S, Eubanks TR, Jacobsen G, et al. Repair of paraesophageal hernias. Am J Surg 1999;177(5):354–8.

37. Treacy PJ, Jamieson GG. An approach to the management of para-oesophageal hiatus hernias. Aust N Z J Surg 1987;57(11):813–7.

38. Rattner DW, Evans NR. Management of minimally symptomatic giant paraesophageal hernias. In: Ferguson MK, editor. Difficult decisions in thoracic surgery: an evidence-based approach. 1st edition. London: Springer-Verlag; 2007. p. 350–5.

39. Sihvo EI, Salo JA, Rasanen JV, et al. Fatal complications of adult paraesophageal hernia: a population-based study. J Thorac Cardiovasc Surg 2009;137(2):419–24.

40. Davis SS Jr. Current controversies in paraesophageal hernia repair. Surg Clin North Am 2008;88(5):959–78, vi.

41. Wichterman K, Geha AS, Cahow CE, et al. Giant paraesophageal hiatus hernia with intrathoracic stomach and colon: the case for early repair. Surgery 1979;86(3):497–506.

42. Callendar GG, Ferguson M. Giant paraesophageal hernia: thoracic, open abdominal, or laparoscopic approach. In: Ferguson MK, editor. Difficult decisions in thoracic surgery: an evidence-based approach. 1st edition. London: Springer-Verlag; 2007. p. 434–9.

43. Parekh KR, Iannettoni MD. Lengthening gastroplasty for managing giant paraesophageal hernia. In: Ferguson MK, editor. Difficult decisions in thoracic surgery: an evidence-based approach. 1st edition. London: Springer-Verlag; 2007. p. 318–22.

44. Altorki NK, Yankelevitz D, Skinner DB. Massive hiatal hernias: the anatomic basis of repair. J Thorac Cardiovasc Surg 1998;115(4):828–35.

45. Patel HJ, Tan BB, Yee J, et al. A 25-year experience with open primary transthoracic repair of paraesophageal hiatal hernia. J Thorac Cardiovasc Surg 2004;127(3):843–9.

46. Williamson WA, Ellis FH Jr, Streitz JM Jr, et al. Paraesophageal hiatal hernia: is an antireflux procedure necessary? Ann Thorac Surg 1993;56(3):447–51.

47. Myers GA, Harms BA, Starling JR. Management of paraesophageal hernia with a selective approach to antireflux surgery. Am J Surg 1995;170(4):375–80.

48. Low DE, Unger T. Open repair of paraesophageal hernia: reassessment of subjective and objective outcomes. Ann Thorac Surg 2005;80(1):287–94.

49. Martin TR, Ferguson MK, Naunheim KS. Management of giant paraesophageal hernia. Dis Esophagus 1997;10(1):47–50.

50. Cuschieri A, Shimi S, Nathanson LK. Laparoscopic reduction, crural repair, and fundoplication of large hiatal hernia. Am J Surg 1992;163(4):425–30.

51. Karmali S, McFadden S, Mitchell P, et al. Primary laparoscopic and open repair of paraesophageal hernias: a comparison of short-term outcomes. Dis Esophagus 2008;21(1):63–8.

52. Trus TL, Bax T, Richardson WS, et al. Complications of laparoscopic paraesophageal hernia repair. J Gastrointest Surg 1997;1(3):221–8.

53. Wiechmann RJ, Ferguson MK, Naunheim KS, et al. Laparoscopic management of giant paraesophageal herniation. Ann Thorac Surg 2001;71(4): 1080–7.

54. Mattar SG, Bowers SP, Galloway KD, et al. Long-term outcome of laparoscopic repair of paraesophageal hernia. Surg Endosc 2002;16(5):745–9.

55. Pierre AF, Luketich JD, Fernando HC, et al. Results of laparoscopic repair of giant paraesophageal hernias: 200 consecutive patients. Ann Thorac Surg 2002;74(6):1909–16.

56. Jobe BA, Aye RW, Deveney CW, et al. Laparoscopic management of giant type III hiatal hernia and short esophagus: objective follow-up at three years. J Gastrointest Surg 2002;6(2):181–8.

57. Diaz S, Brunt LM, Klingensmith ME, et al. Laparoscopic paraesophageal hernia repair, a challenging operation: medium-term outcome of 116 patients. J Gastrointest Surg 2003;7(1):59–67.

58. Andujar JJ, Papasavas PK, Birdas T, et al. Laparoscopic repair of large paraesophageal hernia is associated with a low incidence of recurrence and reoperation. Surg Endosc 2004;18(3):444–7.

59. Boushey RP, Moloo H, Burpee S, et al. Laparoscopic repair of paraesophageal hernias: a Canadian experience. Can J Surg 2008;51(5):355–60.

60. Rathore MA, Andrabi SI, Bhatti MI, et al. Metaanalysis of recurrence after laparoscopic repair of paraesophageal hernia. JSLS 2007;11(4):456–60.

61. Management of giant paraesophageal hiatal hernia. CTSNet: the CardioThoracic Surgery Network. Available at: http://www.ctsnet.org/portals/thoracic/surveys/surveyresults/survey_results_1008.html. Published July 2008. Accessed February 15, 2009.

62. Lorta-Jacob JL. L'endo-brachyesophage. Ann Chir 1957;11:1247.

63. Ponsky J, Rosen M, Fanning A, et al. Anterior gastropexy may reduce the recurrence rate after laparoscopic paraesophageal hernia repair. Surg Endosc 2003;17(7):1036–41.

64. Gastal OL, Hagen JA, Peters JH, et al. Short esophagus: analysis of predictors and clinical implications. Arch Surg 1999;134(6):633–6.

65. Horvath KD, Swanstrom LL, Jobe BA. The short esophagus: pathophysiology, incidence, presentation, and treatment in the era of laparoscopic antireflux surgery. Ann Surg 2000;232(5):630–40.

66. Hill LD, Gelfand M, Bauermeister D. Simplified management of reflux esophagitis with stricture. Ann Surg 1970;172(4):638–51.

67. Pearson FG, Cooper JD, Patterson GA, et al. Gastroplasty and fundoplication for complex reflux problems: long-term results. Ann Surg 1987; 206(4):473–81.

68. Herbella FA, Del Grande JC, Colleoni R. Short esophagus: literature incidence. Dis Esophagus 2002;15(2):125–31.

69. Urbach DR, Khajanchee YS, Glascow RE, et al. Preoperative determinants of an esophageal lengthening procedure in laparoscopic antireflux surgery. Surg Endosc 2001;15(12):1408–12.

70. Demeester SR, Demeester TR. Editorial comment: the short esophagus: going, going, gone? Surgery 2003;133(4):358–63.

71. Kalloor GJ, Deshpande AH, Collis JL. Observations on oesophageal length. Thorax 1976;31(3):284–8.

72. Gozzetti G, Pilotti V, Spangaro M, et al. Pathophysiology and natural history of acquired short esophagus. Surgery 1987;102(3):507–14.

73. Mittal SK, Awad ZT, Tasset M, et al. The preoperative predictability of the short esophagus in patients with stricture or paraesophageal hernia. Surg Endosc 2000;14(5):464–8.

74. Awad ZT, Mittal SK, Roth TA, et al. Esophageal shortening during the era of laparoscopic surgery. World J Surg 2001;25(5):558–61.

75. Madan AK, Frantzides CK, Patsavas KL. The myth of short esophagus. Surg Endosc 2004;18(1):31–4.

76. Collis JL. An operation for hiatus hernia with short esophagus. Thorax 1957;12(3):181–8.

77. Orringer MB, Orringer JS. The combined Collis-Nissen operation: early assessment of reflux control. Ann Thorac Surg 1982;33(6):534–9.

78. Swanstrom LL, Marcus DR, Galloway GQ. Laparoscopic Collis gastroplasty is the treatment of choice for the shortened esophagus. Am J Surg 1996; 171(5):477–81.

79. Johnson AB, Oddsdottir M, Hunter JG. Laparoscopic Collis gastroplasty and Nissen fundoplication: a new technique for the management of esophageal foreshortening. Surg Endosc 1998; 12(8):1055–60.

80. Pearson FG, Cooper JD, Ilves R, et al. Massive hiatal hernia with incarceration: a report of 53 cases. Ann Thorac Surg 1983;35(1):45–51.

81. Morris-Stiff G, Hassn A. Laparoscopic paraoesophageal hernia repair: fundoplication is not usually indicated. Hernia 2008;12(3):299–302.

82. Ellis FH, Crozier RE, Shea JA. Paraesophageal hiatus hernia. Arch Surg 1986;121(4):416–20.

83. Braslow L. Transverse gastropexy vs Stamm gastrostomy in hiatal hernia. Arch Surg 1987;122(7):851.

84. Lichtenstein IL, Shulman AG, Amid PK, et al. The tension-free hernioplasty. Am J Surg 1989;157(2): 188–93.

85. Hinson EL. Early results with Lichtenstein tension-free hernia repair. Br J Surg 1995;82(3):418–9.

86. Utrera Gonzalez A, de la Portilla de Juan F, Carranza Albarran G. Large incisional hernia repair using intraperitoneal placement of expanded polytetrafluoroethylene. Am J Surg 1999;177(4):291–3.

87. Galvani CA, Horgan S. Optimal crural closure techniques for repair of large hiatal hernia. In: Ferguson MK, editor. Difficult decisions in thoracic surgery: an evidence-based approach. 1st edition. London: Springer-Verlag; 2007. p. 371–8.

88. Granderath FA, Kamolz T, Schweiger UM, et al. Impact of laparoscopic Nissen fundoplication with prosthetic hiatal closure on esophageal body motility: results of a prospective randomized trial. Arch Surg 2006;141(7):625–32.

89. Frantzides CT, Madan AK, Carlson MA, et al. A prospective, randomized trial of laparoscopic polytetrafluoroethylene (PTFE) patch repair vs simple cruroplasty for large hiatal hernia. Arch Surg 2002;137(6):649–52.

90. Basso N, De LA, Genco A, et al. 360 degrees laparoscopic fundoplication with tension-free hiatoplasty in the treatment of symptomatic gastroesophageal reflux disease. Surg Endosc 2000; 14(2):164–9.

91. Arendt T, Stuber E, Monig H, et al. Dysphagia due to transmural migration of surgical material into the esophagus nine years after Nissen fundoplication. Gastrointest Endosc 2000;51(5):607–10.

92. Coluccio G, Ponzio S, Ambu V, et al. Dislocation into the cardial lumen of a PTFE prosthesis used in the treatment of voluminous hiatal sliding hernia: a case report. Minerva Chir 2000;55(5): 341–5 [in Italian].

93. Hergueta-Delgado P, Marin-Moreno M, Morales-Conde S, et al. Transmural migration of a prosthetic mesh after surgery of a paraesophageal hiatal hernia. Gastrointest Endosc 2006;64(1):120.

94. Tatum RP, Shalhub S, Oelschlager BK, et al. Complications of PTFE mesh at the diaphragmatic hiatus. J Gastrointest Surg 2008;12(5):953–7.

95. Badylak S, Kokini K, Tullius B, et al. Strength over time of a resorbable bioscaffold for body wall repair in a dog model. J Surg Res 2001;99(2):282–7.

96. Gloeckner DC, Sacks MS, Billiar KL, et al. Mechanical evaluation and design of a multilayered collagenous repair biomaterial. J Biomed Mater Res 2000;52(2):365–73.

97. Hui TT, Thoman DS, Spyrou M, et al. Mesh crural repair of large paraesophageal hiatal hernias. Am Surg 2001;67(12):1170–4.

98. Champion JK, Rock D. Laparoscopic mesh cruroplasty for large paraesophageal hernias. Surg Endosc 2003;17(4):551–3.

99. Keidar A, Szold A. Laparoscopic repair of paraesophageal hernia with selective use of mesh. Surg Laparosc Endosc Percutan Tech 2003;13(3): 149–54.

100. Oelschlager BK, Pellegrini CA, Hunter J, et al. Biologic prosthesis reduces recurrence after laparoscopic paraesophageal hernia repair: a multicenter, prospective, randomized trial. Ann Surg 2006;244(4):481–90.

Acute Traumatic Diaphragmatic Injury

Waël C. Hanna, MD, MBA, Lorenzo E. Ferri, MD, PhD, FRCSC, FACS*

KEYWORDS

- Diaphragm • Trauma • Surgery • Laparoscopy • Flail chest

In 1579, the French military surgeon Ambroise Paré first described the death of a patient from colonic strangulation in a diaphragmatic hernia caused by a remote gunshot wound to the chest. Traumatic diaphragmatic injury still represents an important consequence of penetrating and blunt thoracoabdominal trauma.

INCIDENCE

Although traumatic diaphragmatic injury has been reported in 0.5% to 1.6% of patients hospitalized for blunt trauma,[1] the precise incidence of this injury is likely higher than that reported in these historical series. Diaphragmatic injuries, in the absence of acute diaphragmatic hernias, are often missed by diagnostic imaging and are notoriously underreported. Shah and colleagues[2] report that up to 8% of all patients undergoing a laparotomy or a thoracotomy for trauma will have an incidental finding of diaphragmatic injury.

In a series published in 2008, the authors reported on 105 patients with traumatic diaphragmatic injury out of 24,700 (0.52%) admissions to a level 1 trauma center during a 13-year period. Of those cases, only 44% were associated with a traumatic hernia.[3] With penetrating trauma, the resulting diaphragmatic defect is often too small for herniation in the acute setting. Consequently, acute hernias are present in only one-third of cases under these circumstances. However, with time, an unrecognized diaphragmatic defect may enlarge and, coupled with the gradient between the negative intrathoracic pressure and positive intraabdominal pressure, result in subsequent herniation of intraabdominal contents into the chest. A past history of penetrating thoracoabdominal trauma is not uncommon in patients who present with chronic traumatic hernias[4] (see the article in this issue). On the other hand, with blunt trauma, diaphragmatic injury is a result of dissipation of significant energy from the abdominopelvic cavity into the chest. Hence, traumatic diaphragmatic injuries due to blunt trauma result in a much larger diaphragmatic defect than that seen in penetrating trauma and in a higher rate of herniation.[3,5]

CHARACTERISTICS

Diaphragmatic injury occurs more commonly in the left hemidiaphragm. About 75% of all acute diaphragmatic hernias are encountered in the left chest.[6] Although some authors maintain that the left hemidiaphragm is congenitally weaker at its points of embryonic fusion,[7] it is more likely that the cushioning effect of the liver protects a large portion of the right hemidiaphragm,[8] thus reducing the risk of injury and herniation in this location. Thus, abdominal organs lying to the left of the midline are the ones most frequently found herniating into the chest. The stomach is the organ with the highest rate of involvement in acute hernias (48%), followed by the spleen (26%) and the small bowel, large bowel, and omentum (13%).[3] Although less frequent, right diaphragmatic injuries resulting in herniation of the liver are seen in cases of significant intraabdominal pressure, such as a crush or deceleration injury, resulting in either complete rupture or avulsion of the diaphragm.

By virtue of its location between the chest and abdomen, the diaphragm is rarely injured in isolation. Most acute traumatic diaphragmatic injuries are accompanied by injuries to other organs, with

Division of Thoracic Surgery, McGill University, The Montreal General Hospital, Room L9-112, 1650 Cedar Avenue, Montreal, Quebec, H3G 1A4, Canada
* Corresponding author.
E-mail address: lorenzo.ferri@muhc.mcgill.ca (L.E. Ferri).

Thorac Surg Clin 19 (2009) 485–489
doi:10.1016/j.thorsurg.2009.07.008
1547-4127/09/$ – see front matter © 2009 Elsevier Inc. All rights reserved.

some investigators reporting an incidence of associated injuries as high as 100% and an average Injury Severity Score of 36.[9] The high energy associated with blunt traumatic diaphragmatic injury results in pelvic and long bone fractures in approximately 60% of cases.[10] Traumatic brain injury is present in half of the cases of blunt diaphragmatic injury and is the only reliable predictor of mortality in such patients.[3]

The pattern of associated injuries in penetrating diaphragmatic hernias is predictably different from that in blunt traumatic diaphragmatic hernias. The authors and other investigators have reported that most associated injuries requiring treatment occur in intraabdominal organs, such as the liver, spleen, stomach, or small bowel, irrespective of the external site of the penetrating wound.[3]

DIAGNOSIS
Physical Signs and Symptoms

Because the signs and symptoms of acute diaphragmatic trauma may often be masked by severe concomitant injuries to other organs, a high index of suspicion is necessary for the clinical diagnosis of this condition. The possibility of a diaphragmatic injury should be considered in the context of rapid deceleration or crush injuries. Conversely, a possible diaphragmatic injury should be considered in patients with minimal symptoms after penetrating trauma to certain locations. External penetrating wounds in the anterior thoracoabdominal area, particularly on the left, should heighten awareness of a possible diaphragmatic injury. Patients with acute diaphragmatic hernia may complain of shoulder pain, epigastric pain, vomiting, or shortness of breath. On physical examination, the physician might note the presence of bowel sounds in the chest or the absence of breath sounds because of compression of the lungs by the hernia. Occasionally, a diagnosis of acute traumatic hernia may be made by palpating abdominal viscera on placement of a chest tube and rarely by inspection on examination (**Fig. 1**).

Chest Radiograph

The chest radiograph is an integral adjunct in the Advanced Trauma Life Support guidelines for the initial evaluation of the trauma patient, and is often the first clue to the presence of an acute diaphragmatic injury. Subtle signs on the radiograph, such as an obscured diaphragmatic shadow, elevated hemidiaphragm, irregular diaphragmatic contour, or pleural effusion, can suggest injury to the diaphragm.[11] However, all these findings may also be encountered with the atelectasis,

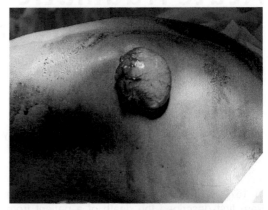

Fig. 1. Penetrating injury to the left lower thorax with obvious herniation of the stomach through the diaphragm and out of the stab wound.

pneumothorax, hemothorax, or pulmonary contusions frequently seen in trauma patients independent of diaphragmatic injury. In the presence of a hernia, a chest radiograph provides the diagnosis in more than 90% of cases.[12] Chest radiography findings consistent with a diaphragmatic hernia include a nasogastric tube coiled in the left chest (stomach in chest) and a supradiaphragmatic air-fluid level (bowel or stomach in chest) (**Fig. 2**). The radiographic findings of a right diaphragmatic injury with herniation of the liver are more subtle, frequently presenting as an elevated hemidiaphragm (**Fig. 3**A). Increasing atelectasis on serial films or an inability to adequately ventilate an intubated patient should also raise the suspicion of a traumatic diaphragmatic hernia. In the

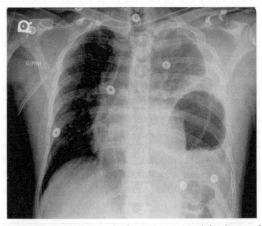

Fig. 2. Chest radiograph depicting typical findings of an acute traumatic diaphragmatic injury with a hernia containing stomach in a patient after a motor vehicle accident. Note the left hemothorax, multiple rib fractures, an air-fluid level, and a curled nasogastric tube in the left chest.

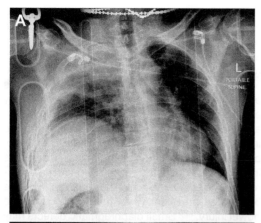

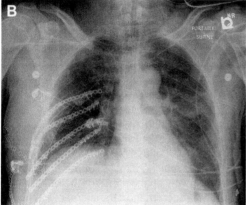

Fig. 3. (*A, B*) Chest radiograph depicting the more subtle signs of an acute right diaphragmatic hernia in a patient sustaining a crush injury. Note the right flail chest and elevated hemidiaphragm typical of a herniated liver (*A*). This patient required internal fixation of the flail segment before placing mattress sutures around the reduced ribs to repair the hernia (*B*).

absence of an acute hernia, the sensitivity of the chest radiograph to diaphragmatic injury is rather limited.[3,13] The authors reported that the trauma bay chest radiograph as read by the emergency physicians detects 23% of diaphragmatic injuries. However, attending radiologists who subsequently read the same images were twice as likely to identify injuries to the diaphragm,[3] suggesting that image interpretation skills need to be improved, taking the above-mentioned signs into consideration.

The use of oral contrast can significantly improve the sensitivity of the chest radiograph for acute diaphragmatic hernias.[14] Although they remain as important diagnostic modalities for chronic diaphragmatic hernias, contrast studies are rarely obtained in the acute setting, where associated injuries may dictate prompt management.

Computed Tomography Scan of the Chest

Computed tomography (CT) scan of the chest has become an essential tool for the evaluation of the hemodynamically stable trauma patient. In the absence of an acute hernia, CT scans offer little benefit compared with conventional plain radiographs, as the sensitivity of CT for the diagnosis of isolated diaphragmatic injury is limited.[15] However, in the presence of herniation of abdominal organs into the thoracic cavity, the sensitivity of oral contrast-enhanced CT scan is close to 95%.[16] The CT scan is especially helpful if the plain chest radiograph is obscured by the presence of a hemothorax or a lung contusion.[14] CT scans offer the luxury of determining which organs have migrated into the chest and may also identify associated injuries. Although some investigators claim that a CT scan can help with operative planning,[16] the authors find that a transabdominal approach is almost universally used in the acute setting, given the high rate of associated intraperitoneal injuries.

Diagnostic Peritoneal Lavage

The sensitivity and specificity of diagnostic peritoneal lavage (DPL) is determined by the red blood cell (RBC) count. A DPL criterion of 1000 RBC/mm^3 has been used to diagnose diaphragm injuries after stab wounds to the lower chest, flank, or back. The appearance of lavage fluid in chest tube drainage is a telltale sign of an injury. However, false-negative results have been noted in 14% to 40% of patients with isolated diaphragmatic injuries in 2 series.[12] The authors have found that DPL is not particularly useful for this condition, and it is included in this article primarily out of historical interest. Furthermore, with the advent of bedside focused assessment with sonography for trauma (FAST), DPL has fallen out of favor and is rarely used, except in the setting where FAST is not available.

Magnetic Resonance Imaging

The utility of magnetic resonance imaging (MRI) for the assessment of diaphragmatic pathology is well recognized. With MRI, in contrast to CT, the diaphragm can be visualized as a discrete structure and hence a rupture of the diaphragm in the absence of a diaphragmatic hernia can often be diagnosed from MRI.[17] However, the use of MRI remains restricted by its limited availability, and more importantly, by its impracticality in the acute setting. Hence, the routine use of MRI in the evaluation of acute diaphragmatic injury is not recommended.

Exploratory Laparoscopy and Thoracoscopy

Noninvasive diagnostic modalities have a very limited sensitivity for diaphragmatic injury in the absence of an obvious diaphragmatic hernia. Thus, in some hemodynamically stable patients who do not require operative intervention to manage associated injuries, there exists a real possibility of missed diaphragmatic injuries, the consequences of which are discussed in Brian Louie's article in this issue. In many centers, the advent of minimally invasive surgical techniques has been used to address this issue. In patients with a high suspicion of diaphragmatic injury, particularly penetrating trauma to the left upper quadrant or left lower chest, the use of exploratory laparoscopy or thoracoscopy has been advocated.[18] Murray and colleagues[19] used exploratory laparoscopy and thoracoscopy and reported an alarming 42% incidence of diaphragmatic injury in patients with penetrating injury to the left thoracoabdominal area. In such situations, the authors prefer to perform a diagnostic laparoscopy to assess the integrity of the diaphragm in patients with penetrating wounds in the left lower chest/left upper quadrant, unless there is a large retained hemothorax necessitating thoracoscopic drainage. Diaphragmatic injuries thus identified can be repaired at the same setting by the minimally invasive approach.

TREATMENT

Acute traumatic diaphragmatic injuries are treated by surgical reduction of the herniated organs, if present, and closure of the diaphragmatic defect. Given the high rate of associated injuries to intraabdominal organs, it is generally recommended to approach the diaphragmatic injury through a midline laparotomy.[3,12] Although penetrating trauma to the chest is often associated with pulmonary injury, surgical intervention other than a chest tube is rarely required. For certain cases in which a thoracotomy is required to manage life-threatening associated injuries, such as ongoing massive hemothorax or aerodigestive tract injury, the diaphragm should be repaired through the chest. Large right diaphragmatic injuries may be difficult to manage through an abdominal approach because of the bulk of the herniated liver and the avulsion of the diaphragmatic attachments to the chest wall and thus necessitate a transthoracic approach. However, in these settings, a simultaneous laparotomy is often indicated to rule out and address possible intraabdominal organ injury.

Two principles must be observed when repairing acute traumatic diaphragmatic hernias: complete reduction of the herniated organs back into the abdomen and watertight closure of the diaphragm to avoid recurrence. Rarely is the hernia difficult to reduce in the acute setting; however, if this is encountered, the phrenotomy can be partially extended to facilitate reduction of a tightly incarcerated herniated organ. Care must be taken not to injure the phrenic nerve in the process. In cases of concomitant perforation of abdominal viscera, it is important to irrigate the chest to reduce the occurrence of an empyema, which has been shown to be 3 times as prevalent when there is documented bowel injury.[3,20] Small diaphragmatic defects may be repaired using interrupted nonabsorbable sutures. Larger defects will require interrupted figure-of-eight or mattress sutures, in either a single layer or a double layer configuration. The authors prefer the use of 0 to 1 nonabsorbable braided sutures for the ease of knot tying. This approach will address most penetrating traumatic injuries to the diaphragm. However, blowout injuries of the diaphragm resulting from high-energy crush or deceleration mechanisms of trauma frequently result in avulsion of this muscle from its chest wall attachments, making simple suture repair impossible, particularly on the right side. In these circumstances, we recommend a transthoracic repair with horizontal mattress sutures to secure the diaphragm around the ribs, recognizing that this may require internal plate and screw fixation of these bones if a large flail segment is present (**Fig. 3**B). Although some investigators have advocated the use of prosthetic mesh to achieve a tension-free repair of large diaphragmatic defects, the authors advise against this approach in the acute setting. The use of prosthetics may be of benefit in the repair of chronic diaphragmatic injury, but it carries a high rate of infection in the acute setting, especially in the presence of hollow viscus injury in the abdomen.

OUTCOMES

Mortality in patients with acute traumatic diaphragmatic injury is entirely dependent on associated injuries and rarely on the diaphragmatic injury itself.[3] Reported mortality rates vary between 18% and 40%, depending on whether the mechanism of trauma is blunt or penetrating.[2,3,18] The most reliable predictor of mortality in patients with an acute diaphragmatic injury is the Injury Severity Score. Other predictors of mortality include high transfusion requirements, rib fractures, and traumatic brain injury, all of which carry severe sequelae and have been shown to be predictors of poor outcome in trauma patients. Long-term follow-up for recurrence after repair of acute traumatic diaphragmatic hernias can be a difficult task. The trauma population tends to be young, mobile, and, especially for those on the receiving end of penetrating trauma, difficult to locate. However, there is a suggestion from our series that the recurrence rate of acute diaphragmatic hernia is higher when absorbable sutures are used for diaphragmatic repair.[3]

SUMMARY

Acute diaphragmatic hernia is a result of diaphragmatic injury that accompanies severe blunt or penetrating thoracoabdominal trauma. It is frequently diagnosed early on the trauma bay chest radiograph or CT scan of the chest. However, in the absence of a hernia, it may be difficult to identify traumatic diaphragmatic injury on conventional imaging. A midline laparotomy is the advocated approach for repair of acute diaphragmatic trauma because it offers the possibility of diagnosing and repairing frequently associated intraabdominal injuries. In hemodynamically stable patients with penetrating left thoracoabdominal trauma, the incidence of injury to the diaphragm is very high, and thoracoscopy or laparoscopy is recommended for the diagnosis and repair of a missed diaphragmatic injury. Repair with nonabsorbable simple sutures is adequate in most cases, and the use of mesh should be reserved for chronic and large defects. Outcomes of acute diaphragmatic hernia repair are largely dictated by the severity of concomitant injuries, with the Injury Severity Score being the most widely recognized predictor of mortality.

REFERENCES

1. Epstein LI, Lempke RE. Rupture of the right hemidiaphragm due to blunt trauma. J Trauma 1968;8:19–28.
2. Shah R, Sabaratnam S, Mearns A. Traumatic rupture of diaphragm. Ann Thorac Surg 1995;60:1444–9.
3. Hanna WC, Ferri LE, Fata P, et al. The current status of traumatic diaphragmatic injury: lessons learned from 105 patients over 13 years. Ann Thorac Surg 2008;85(3):1044–8.
4. Feliciano DV, Cruse PA, Mattox KL, et al. Delayed diagnosis of injuries to the diaphragm after penetrating wounds. J Trauma 1988;28:1135–44.
5. Waldschmidt ML, Laws HL. Injuries of the diaphragm. J Trauma 1980;20:587–91.
6. Schraff JR, Naunheim KS. Traumatic diaphragmatic injuries. Thorac Surg Clin 2007;17:81–5.
7. Andrus CH, Morton JH. Rupture of the diaphragm after blunt trauma. Am J Surg 1970;119:686.
8. Ilgrenfritz SM, Stewart DE. Blunt trauma of the diaphragm. Am J Surg 1992;58:334–9.
9. Ward RE, Flynn TC, Clark WP. Diaphragmatic disruption due to blunt abdominal trauma. J Trauma 1981;21:35–8.
10. Rodriguez-Morales G, Rodriguez A, Shatney CH. Acute rupture of the diaphragm in blunt trauma: analysis of 60 patients. J Trauma 1986;26:438.
11. Carter BN, Guiseffi J, Felson B. Traumatic diaphragmatic hernia. Am J Roentgenol Radium Ther 1951;65:56.
12. Payne JH, Yellin AE. Traumatic diaphragmatic hernia. Arch Surg 1982;117:18.
13. Demetriades D, Kakoyiannis S, Parekh D, et al. Penetrating injuries of the diaphragm. Br J Surg 1988;75:824.
14. Rosati C. Acute traumatic injury to the diaphragm. Chest Surg Clin N Am 1998;8:371–9.
15. Chen JC, Wilson SE. Diaphragmatic injuries: recognition and management in 62 patients. Am Surg 1991;57:810.
16. Marts B, Durham R, Shapiro M, et al. Computed tomography in the diagnosis of blunt thoracic injury. Am J Surg 1994;168:688–92.
17. Boulanger BR, Mirvis SE, Rodriguez A. MRI in traumatic diaphragmatic rupture: case reports. J Trauma 1992;32:89.
18. Ochsner MG, Rozycki GS, Lucente F, et al. Prospective evaluation of thoracoscopy for diagnosing diaphragmatic injury in thoraco-abdominal trauma: a preliminary report. J Trauma 1993;34:704–10.
19. Murray JA, Demetriades D, Cornwell EE III, et al. Penetrating left thoracoabdominal trauma: the incidence and clinical presentation of diaphragm injuries. J Trauma 1997;43(4):624–6.
20. Eren S, Esme H, Sehitogullari A, et al. The risk factors and management of posttraumatic empyema in trauma patients. Injury 2008;39(1):44–9.

Chronic Traumatic Diaphragmatic Hernia

Maurice Blitz, MD, MSc, FRCS(C),
Brian E. Louie, MD, MPH, FRCS(C)*

KEYWORDS

• Trauma • Diaphragm • Hernia • Injury • Chronic

Knowledge of the existence of traumatic diaphragmatic hernias (TDH) has been around for over 500 years. Yet, one of the persistent challenges of studying TDH is that the term encompasses a spectrum of disease based on a temporal pattern ranging from acute to chronic. A TDH may be classified as chronic mere days after the acute event if the original injuries have resolved or may not become apparent until several decades later. The first description of a TDH was by Sennertus[1] in 1541 who reported on a soldier with stomach herniating into his chest 7 months after having sustained the injury: a chronic TDH.

Over the years, much attention has been directed towards TDH. Many of the treatises written have dealt primarily with acute TDH. The entity of chronic TDH has been much less frequently discussed and often lumped in with the management of acute TDH or relegated to a small paragraph at the end of a chapter. This lack of attention is somewhat surprising given the potential for great morbidity and mortality associated with this condition. In 1579, Ambroise Paré described a fatality caused by a strangulated gangrenous colon that had herniated through a small posttraumatic diaphragmatic defect 8 months after the injury was sustained.[2] This article discusses chronic TDH in its definition and epidemiology; the natural history and presentation; the appropriate investigations used to diagnose TDH; and finally, the different methods of treatment and the controversies therein.

DEFINITION

By definition, a traumatic diaphragmatic hernia is the incursion into the thorax of normally intraperitoneal structures after a traumatic event. Many similar terms have been used to describe this event including diaphragmatic rupture, injury, and hernia. The confusion surrounding these incursions relates to how the temporal descriptors are applied to this disease process. The use of acute and chronic to temporally define diaphragmatic hernia has been inconsistent. In some series, acute is defined as the appearance of the herniated viscus within 7 days of the inciting event, while others have used 1 month as the cut off. This definition was arbitrarily decided and applied without regard for whether patients were initially operatively explored or not, whether patients had already been discharged from hospital, or whether the original injuries had resolved.

The most useful classification system was devised by Grimes and was based upon a similar schema devised by Carter and colleagues[3] over 20 years earlier. This definition divides TDH on a temporal basis into three categories: acute, latent, and obstructive.[4] The acute phase starts at the time of the original trauma and continues until the apparent recovery from the injuries incurred. This recovery then signifies the beginning of the latent phase during which patients may or may not be symptomatic. The obstructive phase begins when the herniated viscus becomes incarcerated, potentially leading to ischemia, necrosis or perforation. For the purposes of this discussion,

Division of Thoracic Surgery, Swedish Medical Center, Suite 850, 1101 Madison Street, Seattle, WA 98104, USA
* Corresponding author. Division of Thoracic Surgery, Swedish Medical Center, Suite 850, 1101 Madison Street, Seattle, WA 98104.
E-mail address: brian.louie@swedish.org (B.E. Louie).

Thorac Surg Clin 19 (2009) 491–500
doi:10.1016/j.thorsurg.2009.08.001

a chronic TDH will refer to patients in the latent and obstructive phases (ie, any traumatic diaphragmatic defect recognized after the inevitable accompanying acute traumatic injuries are healed).

EPIDEMIOLOGY AND MECHANISMS OF INJURY

It is very difficult, if not impossible, to ascertain the true incidence, prevalence, and distribution of chronic TDH. The development of a chronic traumatic hernia is directly related to the difficulty of diagnosing an acute diaphragmatic hernia, thus making chronic TDH a direct sequelae of an injury missed during the treatment of an acute traumatic event. An amalgamation of available data suggests that up to 20% of all truncal trauma results in an associated acute TDH.[5–8] However, there is no accurate method to determine which of these acute TDH will go on to become chronic TDH. Some of them will be repaired immediately during the acute phase, some will not be recognized only to become apparent in the future, and some will never be detected. Therefore, it is likely that there are many chronic TDH that are never recognized and never come to clinical attention in any way.

It is informative to separate chronic TDH by mechanism of injury: those resulting from penetrating trauma versus those resulting from blunt trauma.

Penetrating Trauma

The reported incidence of diaphragmatic injury varies from 3.4% to 47% of penetrating thoracoabdominal trauma. Of these patients, 7% to 26% did not have any recognized preoperative indications of TDH aside from the initial history of penetrating trauma.[8–11] Historically, penetrating trauma led to operative exploration or intervention, which led to an increase in the recognition of diaphragmatic involvement in the acute setting. Consequently, this recognition has resulted in less chronic TDH. This statement may no longer hold true as trauma surgery has gravitated towards more aggressive nonoperative management of penetrating trauma. As penetrating injuries are mostly caused by knife wounds, the actual diaphragmatic disruption and tissue loss incurred is often quite small.

In penetrating trauma, the location of injuries is related to the penetrating object and is largely independent of the victim. This independence is reflected in some series that have described an equivalent distribution between right- and left-sided diaphragm injuries.[12,13] There is, however, a pragmatic view that suggests that the right

handedness of the majority of the population leads to a greater preponderance of left-sided penetrating knife trauma and thereby proportionally more left-sided TDH caused by penetrating trauma.[14] Confusing things further, the liver may mask small right-sided injuries from being discovered.

Blunt Trauma

In blunt abdominal or thoracic trauma, the overall incidence of TDH has been reported to be 0.8% to 20%.[5–8] Historically, 33% to 67% of these diaphragmatic injuries were missed acutely[7,15–20] in part because of the distraction caused by the severity of the patients' associated injuries (up to 94%–100%[7,21]) and their treatment. Before the advent of sophisticated imaging, such as ultrasound and helical CT, early operative management of blunt trauma patients was standard. This standardization led to a decrease in the incidence of delayed diagnosis of traumatic diaphragmatic hernia.[22] Most recently, the pendulum has swung toward nonoperative management for blunt traumatic injuries, which may be resulting in an increase in missed diaphragmatic injuries and therefore an increase in chronic TDH.[23]

Unlike in penetrating trauma, the diaphragmatic injuries resulting from blunt trauma are unevenly distributed: 50% to 80% are isolated to the left hemidiaphragm, 12% to 40% to the right hemidiaphragm, and 1% to 9% are reported to be bilateral.[12,21,24–32] Many theories exist for why there may be a predilection for left-sided injuries. The most dominant theory is that the liver is protective, directly and indirectly, as it dissipates some of the traumatic forces.[33,34] This distribution is refuted by an autopsy series of 171 blunt trauma victims that demonstrated that there was no predilection for left-sided injuries over right.[35] These differing conclusions may be reconciled by the explanation that there is an increased likelihood of fatality with blunt trauma when the forces are great enough to injure the right diaphragm and the liver. This likelihood decreases the number of surviving trauma victims with right-sided TDH, leaving the preponderance of the hernias left sided.

The most common site of injury in blunt trauma involves the inherently weak area where the lumbar and costal leaflets of the diaphragm fuse during embryological development. Left-sided injuries are therefore predominantly posterolateral and tend to extend radially and medially towards the central tendon.[15,36] Because of the tremendous force needed to cause this injury, they tend to result in greater tissue defects than do those caused by penetrating trauma (**Fig. 1**).

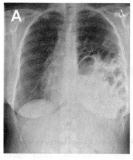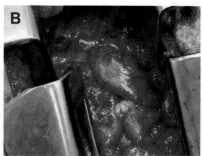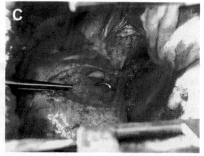

Fig. 1. Chronic Traumatic Diaphragmatic Hernia. (*A*) Plain CXR demonstrating chronic TDH with associated viscus in the left hemithorax. (*B*) Low posterolateral thoracotomy demonstrating small bowel, large bowel, and liver tip inside left hemithorax. (*C*) Once hernia has been reduced, resultant diaphragmatic defect is demonstrated.

Iatrogenic Injury

A variant of the traumatic chronic diaphragmatic hernia are those that result from iatrogenic injury. These injuries are rarely studied but often cited as a potential cause of TDH. They may result from direct diaphragmatic injury (chest tube through diaphragm, purposeful takedown of diaphragm with attempted reconstruction) or indirect diaphragmatic injury (retraction, cautery arc, cryoablation injury).

NATURAL HISTORY OF DIAPHRAGMATIC INJURY

Acute diaphragmatic defects can vary in size, from barely large enough to fit a finger to massive tissue loss creating defects greater than 10 cm in size. The exact natural history of these injuries is unknown. It is possible that some penetrating injuries from small caliber weapons may heal without surgical intervention and remain clinically quiescent throughout patients' lives. For most injuries, progressive enlargement of the injury site is likely.

The development of clinically symptomatic, if not life threatening, chronic TDH from an initially small and unrecognized acute TDH may be at least partially caused by the physiology of the abdomen and chest. The chest's negative intrapleural pressure effectively pulls intra-abdominal contents upwards through any diaphragmatic defect, while the positive intra-abdominal pressure pushes these contents in the same direction. There is normally a gradient of 7 to 10 cm H_2O effecting this process. This gradient can increase dramatically during deep inspiration, coughing, or pregnancy and has been reported to reach up to 100 cm H_2O.[37,38] In addition, there are radial forces constantly placed on the diaphragm by the act of respiration that may distract the tissue edges at the site of injury.

The combination of the two forces results in the progressive enlargement of the diaphragmatic defect and displacement of the intra-abdominal contents into the chest. Many different herniating tissues have been described, including omentum, stomach, colon, small bowel, spleen, and rarely kidney in left-sided chronic TDH, and liver, colon, small bowel, and omentum in right-sided chronic TDH. Multiple organs can, and often are, involved in a single hernia. When enough normally subdiaphragmatic tissue has been displaced into the chest, patients may begin to experience symptoms. As the diaphragmatic defect increases in size, the contribution of the involved hemidiaphragm tends to decrease, thereby affecting pulmonary function. This effect may be initially demonstrated by decreased exercise tolerance and can progress to frank dyspnea at rest. These respiratory effects may then be compounded by the impediment to lung expansion created by the abdominal viscera occupying intrathoracic space. With continued displacement of more viscera, the mediastinum may slowly shift to the contralateral chest leading to impairment of venous return, thereby exaggerating symptoms further.[39] This entire process may last days to years and represents the latent phase as described earlier.

The cause of major morbidity and mortality in chronic TDH occurs when patients enter the obstructive phase, which is related to the interaction between the diaphragmatic defect and the specific viscera that have herniated into the chest. With larger defects, herniation of a hollow viscus may lead to volvulus, whereas strangulation and perforation are more likely in patients who have large volumes of tissue herniating through smaller defects.

PRESENTATION

The presentation of patients who have chronic TDH varies widely. Sometimes chronic TDH is detected incidentally on imaging for nonrelated reasons. In these patients, a careful history of, often very remote, antecedent trauma is then needed to make the diagnosis. Symptomatology may be related to the gastrointestinal (GI) tract, the respiratory tract, or be one of nonspecific pain (**Box 1**). These symptoms are reflective of viscera having herniated into the chest or occupying space within the thoracic cavity. Most dramatically, some patients present in extremis because of severe complications from their hernia. These complications include direct gastrointestinal effects, such as complete obstruction, ischemia, and perforation of hollow viscus.[40] The rapid expansion of herniated viscus may also lead to significant respiratory and cardiovascular effects that can mimic a tension pneumothorax.[37,41,42]

DIAGNOSIS

The diagnosis of chronic TDH is generally determined by a history identifying a previous episode of trauma and imaging confirming the presence of intra-abdominal contents within the thoracic cavity.

History

A key and necessary feature in making the diagnosis of chronic TDH is an antecedent history of blunt or penetrating trauma. This history may be difficult to elicit as the trauma may be quite remote. There are reports of patients presenting with chronic TDH as many as 50 years after the likely occurrence of the initial diaphragmatic injury.[43,44] Symptomatology is varied in timing of onset, type, severity, and position. The potentially late onset of symptoms attributable to TDH, therefore, often impedes making an early diagnosis. In the latent stage, if symptomatic, patients are much more likely to have innocuous, and thereby, easily missed symptoms (see **Box 1**). These vague symptoms can lead to the incorrect diagnosis of peptic ulcer disease or gallbladder disease. As patients become more symptomatic, they may present with acute respiratory deterioration, such as dyspnea, profound tachycardia, and even cyanosis. These symptoms may be separate from, or in conjunction with, severe pain and gastrointestinal hemorrhage.[25]

Physical Examination

Unfortunately, the physical examination is not often helpful in making the diagnosis of chronic TDH. In the latent phase, the exam will either be entirely normal or there will be subtle signs, such as decreased air entry on the affected side or bowel sounds over the hemithorax. In the obstructive phase, the physical examination reflects the systemic effects of the compromised viscera, which may include fever and tachycardia along with a history of increasing pain. In addition, signs of dehydration may also be present if the herniated viscus is obstructed. Once these signs are recognized, treatment should be redirected to focus on resuscitation and rapid definitive treatment of patients.

Radiology

Chest X rays
A sizeable proportion of the relevant literature comments on the utility of chest X rays (CXR) in acute TDH. In that body of literature, the described diagnostic utility of the plain chest X ray is limited, with only 25% to 49% of initial chest X rays being of diagnostic value.[45] These numbers may be increased if the films are serially repeated or if adjuncts, such as nasogastric (NG) tubes, or contrast dyes are used. Although the diagnostic accuracy may not be applicable to chronic TDH, the specific radiologic findings are generalizable. Specific signs include identifying the presence of abdominal viscera within the chest, possibly in conjunction with the collar sign, which is identified as the appearance of focal constriction at the site where the viscera traverse the diaphragmatic breach. Identification of the NG tip within the left hemithorax is also indicative of diaphragmatic injury (**Fig. 2**). CXR is less helpful in the setting of right-sided TDH as it is much less common for hollow viscera to herniate into this hemithorax largely because of the obstructive presence of

---

Box 1
Most common presenting symptoms

Gastrointestinal

   Nausea

   Vomiting

   Early satiety

   Pain (postprandial)

   Intermittent (partial) obstructive symptoms

Pulmonary

   Shortness of breath on exertion

   Shortness of breath

   Decreased exercise tolerance

General

   Chest or abdominal pain/discomfort

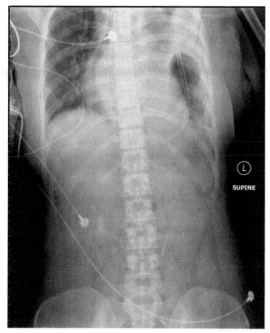

Fig. 2. Plain radiograph demonstrating NG with distal end in supradiaphragmatic position secondary to a chronic TDH.

the liver. In addition, the contour of liver itself mimics the diaphragmatic shadow and may be difficult, if not impossible, to differentiate from normal diaphragm. Less sensitive, but suggestive, signs particular to right-sided TDH include diaphragmatic elevation with mediastinal shift and obscuration of the diaphragmatic margin.

CT

Initially CT scanning was only marginally better than X rays in detecting TDH, but the introduction of helical CT scanners has demonstrated greatly improved sensitivity (71%–100%) and specificity (75%–100%). These values differ between right and left TDH, with improved detection on the left.[46–48] These already acceptable results should continue to improve as multidetector scanners allow increased resolution while decreasing slice thickness.[49] The improvement in detection using the CT scanner is not only because of the increasingly higher resolution offered but also because of the ability to reformat images into coronal and sagittal views. The use of multiple planes has allowed, with increasing precision, the identification of the exact site of rupture on the diaphragm.

Using the images generated by the CT scan, there are numerous ways to detect TDH. Direct visualization of the injury and nonvisualization of portions of the diaphragm indicates a breach. This is breach is also indicated by the presence

of herniated viscera within the thorax. Indirect signs include the collar sign as described in plain radiographs (**Fig. 3**) and the dependent viscera sign. In supine patients, normally the intra-abdominal viscera are removed from the posterior chest wall by the diaphragm. In cases where there is a disruption in the diaphragmatic fibers, the viscera are no longer constrained and may abut the posterior chest wall. In right-sided tears this can result in the liver lying directly against the posterior chest wall, while in left-sided injuries one may see the spleen abutting the posterior chest wall. Alternatively, a variation includes visualizing the bowel posterior to the spleen.[50]

MRI

Although the use of MRI has largely been panned in the acute setting because of time and logistical factors, it is potentially of great benefit to those presenting in the latent phase with chronic TDH. Using T1 weighted imaging, this modality is able to clearly differentiate diaphragm from adjacent tissues, such as lung or liver, and thereby demonstrate diaphragmatic defects and tissues protruding through them.[50,51] Like CT, the ability to view in the sagittal and coronal planes is greatly beneficial because it allows recognition of the site of rupture. With the advent of multiplanar reconstruction on CT, the utility of MRI has begun to wane.

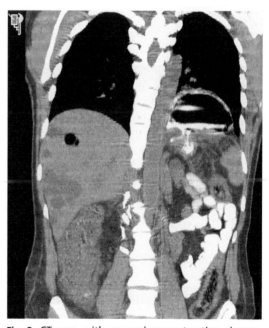

Fig. 3. CT scan with coronal reconstruction demonstrating collar sign.

Contrast radiography

In many centers the use of CT has replaced formal GI fluoroscopy in the diagnosis of TDH. However, the demonstration of oral, and occasionally rectal, contrast in a gas containing viscus within the thoracic cavity is diagnostic of a TDH (**Fig. 4**).

Nuclear medicine/ultrasonography

Nuclear medicine imaging and ultrasound have very limited roles in the diagnosis of chronic TDH. Historically, nuclear medicine imaging in the form of radionuclide hepatobiliary scans (ie, 99mTc scintigraphy) had been used occasionally to aid in detecting supradiaphragmatic liver segments.[52] This technique was used because of the added difficulty caused by potential hepatic involvement in right-sided TDH. This difficulty was attributable to the inability to consistently distinguish between liver protruding through the diaphragm, normal diaphragmatic dome, and sub-diaphragmatic liver. A second nuclear medicine study, the spleen scan, has been advocated in left-side TDH with pleural nodules seen on CT, as these may represent splenosis.[53,54] Ultrasound has also been used to look at diaphragmatic motion. Although potentially useful, it is severely limited by aerated lung and intraluminal air in viscera. Except in specific clinical situations, nuclear medicine and ultrasonographic studies, like most other radiological investigations, have been supplanted by increasingly sensitive multidetector CT scanners.

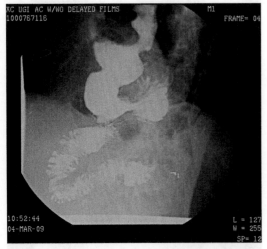

XC UGI AC W/WO DELAYED FILMS   M1
1000767116   FRAME= 04

10:52:44
04-MAR-09   L = 127
                                     W = 255
                                     SP= 12

Fig. 4. Small bowel follow through demonstrating small bowel herniating into left chest by way of chronic TDH.

Diagnostic procedures

Thoracoscopy and laparoscopy have a very limited role in the diagnosis of chronic TDH. Thoracoscopy has been advocated in the acute setting with a diagnostic sensitivity and specificity approaching 100%.[55] In the chronic setting, however, laparoscopy has been advocated when all other diagnostic tests have failed to demonstrate the defect and hernia.[56] Caution must be exercised when this is used because of the potential for creating a pneumothorax through insufflation of the abdomen. Diagnostic thoracoscopy may be beneficial when patients have had major intra-abdominal injuries managed by laparotomy and the potential for adhesions is significant, or in highly selected cases, where the lesion cannot be distinguished from eventration or the dome of the liver by imaging.

MANAGEMENT

Making the diagnosis of a chronic TDH is an indication for operative repair for all patients without prohibitive underlying medical conditions. The urgency and immediacy of proceeding to the operating room depends on the patient and the symptoms. For patients in the latent phase, elective repair of the hernia usually can proceed without further investigations. For patients in the obstructive phase who have presumed gastric herniation, placement of a NG tube to allow decompression of a herniated stomach prior to induction of anesthesia may avoid the potential problem of gastric overdistension with cardiopulmonary compression and aspiration. In the authors' experience, patients who are obstructed and who have systemic signs suggestive of incarceration or impending strangulation can, at times, be converted from an emergent case to an urgent case with judicious endoscopy to evaluate the mucosa of the herniated viscus for ischemia, nasogastric decompression, and aggressive resuscitation.

Operative Approaches

Traditionally, chronic TDH has been approached transabdominally or transthoracically and in recent years has also been undertaken minimally invasively with the laparoscope or thoracoscope. The authors favor an open transthoracic approach for the majority of cases, but acknowledge that there is controversy surrounding the choice of access. That choice is related to the surgical subspecialty of the surgeon, with general surgeons opting for significantly more laparotomies, whereas thoracic surgeons favor thoracotomy in the majority of cases.[12,21,57] Advocates of both approaches agree that in certain clinical circumstances, the addition of a second incision into the alternate cavity or extension of the original incision into the other cavity may be needed to complete the procedure safely and effectively.

Transthoracic Approach

In the authors' experience, an open transthoracic approach offers the most flexibility in the treatment of chronic TDH whether patients present in the latent or obstructive phase. A standard seventh or eighth interspace thoracotomy provides excellent visualization and access to the diaphragm; allows for the repair of the diaphragm and definitive treatment of any obstructive complications, such as perforation; and, if needed, allows for improved access to the abdominal organs by extending the incision across the costal arch (thoracoabdominal incision)[26,58,59] by adding a laparotomy or by incising the diaphragm circumferentially 1 to 2 cm from the edge. It is also preferred because of the concerns regarding adhesions of the herniated tissues to the lung[60] and for right-sided chronic TDH with liver herniation with the possible addition of a right subcostal laparotomy to allow for safe reduction of the liver.[61]

More recently, thoracoscopy has been successfully used in a limited number of elective cases,[62,63] but visualization of the peritoneal cavity and viscera is potentially difficult. This difficulty could potentially lead to missing iatrogenic intraperitoneal injuries. However, as experience grows with minimally invasive thoracic surgery, more cases, specifically those in the latent phase, may be deemed amenable to attempted thoracoscopic intervention. If this is being done, one must not hesitate to convert to open thoracotomy when needed to perform a safe and adequate repair.

Transabdominal Approach

There are many descriptions within the literature regarding transabdominal approaches, open and laparoscopic, being successfully and safely used in the operative management of chronic TDH.[19,59,64,65] The transabdominal approach is often considered less attractive because of the difficulty in addressing the adhesive component to the lung and other thoracic structures, which can reach the upper aspect of the chest, although several recent reports describe the successful transabdominal management of a chronic TDH.[19,59,64,65] Adhesions in the abdomen caused by the severe trauma that was needed to create the diaphragmatic defect may also be formidable. The options for accessing the chest, if necessary, without changing the position of patients are also

less attractive. Although an anterolateral thoracotomy can provide access to the chest, it is limited in viewing the posterior aspect of the chest where the dependent viscera may be adherent. In these cases, closure of the laparotomy and repositioning of patients to proceed with a standard low-posterolateral thoracotomy to complete the repair is preferred.

Although the minimally invasive approach seems to be increasing in popularity, this technique has also been associated with specific and unique complications. Described complications of the laparoscopic approach include pneumothorax and its concomitant cardiovascular effects, which can be avoided by the placement of a chest tube prior to insufflation of the peritoneal cavity.[66] Gas embolization is also a potential complication. Those advocating a minimally invasive approach do endorse that certain injuries, such as those extending to or through the esophageal hiatus or those associated with defects greater than or equal to 10 cm, may be better approached using an open approach.[19]

Operative Technique

The authors prefer a seventh or eighth interspace posterolateral thoracotomy to establish access to the chest. Careful dissection is used to completely free the herniated structures from the thoracic contents and allowing their reduction through the diaphragmatic defect into the peritoneal cavity. The undersurface of the diaphragmatic defect is then freed circumferentially. When completed, the edges are brought together to evaluate for tension. If the edges easily approximate, the authors perform a primary closure with interrupted 0 Ethibond (Ethicon Inc, Somerville, NJ) horizontal mattress sutures that are placed under direct visualization followed by a running, locked #1 Prolene (Ethicon Inc, Somerville, NJ) placed along the tissue ridge resulting from the mattress sutures. Although many different methods have been published, the sole aspect that appears consistent is the use of large (ie, 0 or >) and long-lasting or permanent suture.[7,12,21,26,57,67] A single basal chest tube is placed along the diaphragm.

Many different prostheses, such as mersilene mesh, polytetrafluoroethylene (PTFE), Duo-mesh, polypropylene or polydioxanone patches, have been used successfully in these repairs.[19,58,61,68–71] The authors' goal is to have a tension-free repair, so they tend to err on the side of using mesh to avoid tension. If there is significant tension on the edges sometimes indicated by flattening the diaphragm, or a defect is so large that re-approximation is not feasible, the authors use prosthetic material.

Similarly, if suture tension is so great as to suggest the need for pledgets, the authors will employ a prosthesis rather than place pledgets to absorb the tension. It is the authors' preference to use 2 mm PTFE patches when a prosthesis is required as they believe it prevents transdiaphragmatic fluid shifts, is resistant to adhesion formation, and is robust.

MORBIDITY AND MORTALITY

In chronic TDH, the morbidity and mortality of surgical intervention varies dramatically between those treated in the latent stage and those in the obstructive stage at the time of surgery. In the latent stage, perioperative mortality less than 10% should be expected.[6,40,72] This percentage largely reflects the morbidity inherent in the approach used and the patients' own comorbidities without much affect from the hernia repair itself. In contrast, much greater morbidity (>60%) and mortality (25%–80%) is reported for those presenting with obstructive symptoms and complications from chronic TDH.[20,24,40] These values reinforce the need to pursue the diagnosis in an attempt to make it early, thereby avoiding much of this increased morbidity and mortality.

SUMMARY

Chronic traumatic diaphragmatic hernia is an uncommon but persistent diagnosis associated with significant morbidity and mortality. Chronic TDH describes a spectrum of disease in antecedent mechanism of injury, timing of presentation, size of diaphragmatic defect, and amount and type of tissue displaced into the chest. Multiplanar CT with coronal, sagittal, and axial reconstruction is most effective in making this diagnosis. Once diagnosed, repair should be undertaken. Although transabdominal approaches may be successful, the authors prefer an open transthoracic approach, recognizing that either approach may need to incorporate access into the other body cavity to complete the repair. Basic hernia principles apply including the construction of a tension-free repair, which may necessitate the use of prosthetics. As surgeons become increasingly comfortable with minimally invasive techniques, more chronic TDH are likely to be approached in this fashion. Finally, as much of the morbidity and mortality is associated with the catastrophic consequences of chronic TDH, vigilance needs to be applied in an attempt to diagnose and then repair TDH while in the latent stage prior to the development of the catastrophic complications that herald the obstructive stage.

REFERENCES

1. Sennertus RC. Diaphragmatic hernia produced by a penetrating wound. Edinburgh Med Surg J 1840; 53(104). (Cited by Reed).
2. Hanby W. The case reports and autopsy records of Ambroise Pare. Springfield (IL): Thomas; 1968.
3. Carter BN, Giuseffi J, Felson B. Traumatic diaphragmatic hernia. Am J Roentgenol Radium Ther 1951; 65(1):56–72.
4. Grimes OF. Traumatic injuries of the diaphragm. Diaphragmatic hernia. Am J Surg 1974;128(2):175–81.
5. Alyono D, Perry JF Jr. Impact of speed limit. I. Chest injuries, review of 966 cases. J Thorac Cardiovasc Surg 1982;83(4):519–22.
6. de la Rocha AG, Creel RJ, Mulligan GW, et al. Diaphragmatic rupture due to blunt abdominal trauma. Surg Gynecol Obstet 1982;154(2):175–80.
7. Shah R, Sabanathan S, Mearns AJ, et al. Traumatic rupture of diaphragm. Ann Thorac Surg 1995; 60(5):1444–9.
8. Rubikas R. Diaphragmatic injuries. Eur J Cardiothorac Surg 2001;20(1):53–7.
9. Powell BS, Magnotti LJ, Schroeppel TJ, et al. Diagnostic laparoscopy for the evaluation of occult diaphragmatic injury following penetrating thoracoabdominal trauma. Injury 2008;39(5):530–4.
10. Leppaniemi A, Haapiainen R. Occult diaphragmatic injuries caused by stab wounds. J Trauma 2003; 55(4):646–50.
11. Murray JA, Berne J, Asensio JA. Penetrating thoracoabdominal trauma. Emerg Med Clin North Am 1998;16(1):107–28.
12. Mihos P, Potaris K, Gakidis J, et al. Traumatic rupture of the diaphragm: experience with 65 patients. Injury 2003;34(3):169–72.
13. Shanmuganathan K, Killeen K, Mirvis SE, et al. Imaging of diaphragmatic injuries. J Thorac Imaging 2000;15(2):104–11.
14. Tarver RD, Conces DJ Jr, Cory DA, et al. Imaging the diaphragm and its disorders. J Thorac Imaging 1989;4(1):1–18.
15. Lucido JL, Wall CA. Rupture of the diaphragm due to blunt trauma. Arch Surg 1963;86:989–99.
16. Schwindt WD, Gale JW. Late recognition and treatment of traumatic diaphragmatic hernias. Arch Surg 1967;94(3):330–4.
17. Saegesser F, Besson A. [493 open and closed thoracoabdominal or abdomino-thoracic injuries, 114 of them with involvement of the diaphragm. 1956–1975]. Helv Chir Acta 1977;44(1–2):7–48 [in French].
18. McCune RP, Roda CP, Eckert C. Rupture of the diaphragm caused by blunt trauma. J Trauma 1976; 16(7):531–7.
19. Matthews BD, Bui H, Harold KL, et al. Laparoscopic repair of traumatic diaphragmatic injuries. Surg Endosc 2003;17(2):254–8.

20. Payne JH Jr, Yellin AE. Traumatic diaphragmatic hernia. Arch Surg 1982;117(1):18–24.

21. Athanassiadi K, Kalavrouziotis G, Athanassiou M, et al. Blunt diaphragmatic rupture. Eur J Cardiothorac Surg 1999;15(4):469–74.

22. Miller L, Bennett EV Jr, Root HD, et al. Management of penetrating and blunt diaphragmatic injury. J Trauma 1984;24(5):403–9.

23. Ver MR, Rakhlin A, Baccay F, et al. Minimally invasive repair of traumatic right-sided diaphragmatic hernia with delayed diagnosis. JSLS 2007;11(4):481–6.

24. Demetriades D, Kakoyiannis S, Parekh D, et al. Penetrating injuries of the diaphragm. Br J Surg 1988;75(8):824–6.

25. Mitchell DC, Lea RE. Late presentation of diaphragmatic hernia: a missed diagnosis. BMJ 1988;297(6650):734–5.

26. Matsevych OY. Blunt diaphragmatic rupture: four year's experience. Hernia 2008;12(1):73–8.

27. Eren S, Kantarci M, Okur A. Imaging of diaphragmatic rupture after trauma. Clin Radiol 2006;61(6):467–77.

28. Nursal TZ, Ugurlu M, Kologlu M, et al. Traumatic diaphragmatic hernias: a report of 26 cases. Hernia 2001;5(1):25–9.

29. Rodriguez-Morales G, Rodriguez A, Shatney CH. Acute rupture of the diaphragm in blunt trauma: analysis of 60 patients. J Trauma 1986;26(5):438–44.

30. Kearney PA, Rouhana SW, Burney RE. Blunt rupture of the diaphragm: mechanism, diagnosis, and treatment. Ann Emerg Med 1989;18(12):1326–30.

31. Estrera AS, Landay MJ, McClelland RN. Blunt traumatic rupture of the right hemidiaphragm: experience in 12 patients. Ann Thorac Surg 1985;39(6):525–30.

32. Gelman R, Mirvis SE, Gens D. Diaphragmatic rupture due to blunt trauma: sensitivity of plain chest radiographs. AJR Am J Roentgenol 1991;156(1):51–7.

33. Fajolu O. Traumatic diaphragmatic hernia. J Natl Med Assoc 1984;76(12):1163–4.

34. Flancbaum L, Morgan AS, Esposito T, et al. Non-left sided diaphragmatic rupture due to blunt trauma. Surg Gynecol Obstet 1985;161(3):266–70.

35. Puffer P, Gaebler M. [Traumatic diaphragmatic rupture in a forensic medicine autopsy sample]. Beitr Gerichtl Med 1991;49:149–52 [in German].

36. Ward RE, Flynn TC, Clark WP. Diaphragmatic disruption secondary to blunt abdominal trauma. J Trauma 1981;21(1):35–8.

37. Reber PU, Schmied B, Seiler CA, et al. Missed diaphragmatic injuries and their long-term sequelae. J Trauma 1998;44(1):183–8.

38. Waldschmidt ML, Laws HL. Injuries of the diaphragm. J Trauma 1980;20(7):587–92.

39. Beauchamp G, Khalfallah A, Girard R, et al. Blunt diaphragmatic rupture. Am J Surg 1984;148(2):292–5.

40. Degiannis E, Levy RD, Sofianos C, et al. Diaphragmatic herniation after penetrating trauma. Br J Surg 1996;83(1):88–91.

41. Maddox PR, Mansel RE, Butchart EG. Traumatic rupture of the diaphragm: a difficult diagnosis. Injury 1991;22(4):299–302.

42. Seelig MH, Klingler PJ, Schonleben K. Tension fecopneumothorax due to colonic perforation in a diaphragmatic hernia. Chest 1999;115(1):288–91.

43. Faul JL. Diaphragmatic rupture presenting forty years after injury. Injury 1998;29(6):479–80.

44. Singh S, Kalan MM, Moreyra CE, et al. Diaphragmatic rupture presenting 50 years after the traumatic event. J Trauma 2000;49(1):156–9.

45. Nau T, Seitz H, Mousavi M, et al. The diagnostic dilemma of traumatic rupture of the diaphragm. Surg Endosc 2001;15(9):992–6.

46. Killeen KL, Mirvis SE, Shanmuganathan K. Helical CT of diaphragmatic rupture caused by blunt trauma. AJR Am J Roentgenol 1999;173(6):1611–6.

47. Larici AR, Gotway MB, Litt HI, et al. Helical CT with sagittal and coronal reconstructions: accuracy for detection of diaphragmatic injury. AJR Am J Roentgenol 2002;179(2):451–7.

48. Nchimi A, Szapiro D, Ghaye B, et al. Helical CT of blunt diaphragmatic rupture. AJR Am J Roentgenol 2005;184(1):24–30.

49. Rees O, Mirvis SE, Shanmuganathan K. Multidetector-row CT of right hemidiaphragmatic rupture caused by blunt trauma: a review of 12 cases. Clin Radiol 2005;60(12):1280–9.

50. Sliker CW. Imaging of diaphragm injuries. Radiol Clin North Am 2006;44(2):199–211, vii.

51. Mirvis SE, Shanmuganagthan K. Imaging hemidiaphragmatic injury. Eur Radiol 2007;17(6):1411–21.

52. May AK, Moore MM. Diagnosis of blunt rupture of the right hemidiaphragm by technetium scan. Am Surg 1999;65(8):761–5.

53. Khan AM, Manzoor K, Gordon D, et al. Thoracic splenosis: a diagnosis by history and imaging. Respirology 2008;13(3):481–3.

54. Beekman RA, Louie BE, Singh R, et al. Asymptomatic thoracic splenosis after thoracoabdominal trauma: establishing a diagnosis. Injury Extra 2005;36:283–6.

55. Koehler RH, Smith RS. Thoracoscopic repair of missed diaphragmatic injury in penetrating trauma: case report. J Trauma 1994;36(3):424–7.

56. Mansour KA. Trauma to the diaphragm. Chest Surg Clin N Am 1997;7(2):373–83.

57. Haciibrahimoglu G, Solak O, Olcmen A, et al. Management of traumatic diaphragmatic rupture. Surg Today 2004;34(2):111–4.

58. Sattler S, Canty TG Jr, Mulligan MS, et al. Chronic traumatic and congenital diaphragmatic hernias: presentation and surgical management. Can Respir J 2002;9(2):135–9.

59. Murray JA, Weng J, Velmahos GC, et al. Abdominal approach to chronic diaphragmatic hernias: is it safe? Am Surg 2004;70(10):897–900.

60. Kaw LL Jr, Potenza BM, Coimbra R, et al. Traumatic diaphragmatic hernia. J Am Coll Surg 2004;198(4):668–9.

61. Igai H, Yokomise H, Kumagai K, et al. Delayed hepatothorax due to right-sided traumatic diaphragmatic rupture. Gen Thorac Cardiovasc Surg 2007; 55(10):434–6.

62. Kocher TM, Gurke L, Kuhrmeier A, et al. Misleading symptoms after a minor blunt chest trauma. Thoracoscopic treatment of diaphragmatic rupture. Surg Endosc 1998;12(6):879–81.

63. Kurata K, Kubota K, Oosawa H, et al. Thoracoscopic repair of traumatic diaphragmatic rupture. A case report. Surg Endosc 1996;10(8):850–1.

64. Laws HL, Waldschmidt ML. Rupture of diaphragm. JAMA 1980;243(1):32.

65. Huttl TP, Lang R, Meyer G. Long-term results after laparoscopic repair of traumatic diaphragmatic hernias. J Trauma 2002;52(3):562–6.

66. Meyer G, Huttl TP, Hatz RA, et al. Laparoscopic repair of traumatic diaphragmatic hernias. Surg Endosc 2000;14(11):1010–4.

67. Karmy-Jones R, Jurkovich GJ. Blunt chest trauma. Curr Probl Surg 2004;41(3):211–380.

68. Baldassarre E, Valenti G, Gambino M, et al. The role of laparoscopy in the diagnosis and the treatment of missed diaphragmatic hernia after penetrating trauma. J Laparoendosc Adv Surg Tech A 2007; 17(3):302–6.

69. Matz A, Landau O, Alis M, et al. The role of laparoscopy in the diagnosis and treatment of missed diaphragmatic rupture. Surg Endosc 2000;14(6): 537–9.

70. Shah S, Matthews BD, Sing RF, et al. Laparoscopic repair of a chronic diaphragmatic hernia. Surg Laparosc Endosc Percutan Tech 2000;10(3): 182–6.

71. Slim K, Bousquet J, Chipponi J. Laparoscopic repair of missed blunt diaphragmatic rupture using a prosthesis. Surg Endosc 1998;12(11): 1358–60.

72. McElwee TB, Myers RT, Pennell TC. Diaphragmatic rupture from blunt trauma. Am Surg 1984;50(3): 143–9.

Acquired Paralysis of the Diaphragm

Michael Augustine Ko, MD, PhD, Gail Elizabeth Darling, MD*

KEYWORDS

- Diaphragmatic paralysis • Plication
- Phrenic nerve palsy • Dyspnea • Diagnosis

Diaphragmatic paralysis (DP) occurs when traumatic injury, systemic disease, or neurologic process results in the loss of control of the hemidiaphragms. Symptomatology is dependent on whether or not one or both hemidiaphragms are affected, the onset of paralysis, and the presence or absence of underlying pulmonary disease. Patients with severe respiratory derangement may require intermittent continuous positive airway pressure (CPAP) or bilevel positive airway pressure (BiPAP) or even prolonged mechanical ventilation. Less severely symptomatic patients can be managed through a program of respiratory rehabilitation or by operative diaphragmatic plication. Video-assisted techniques for plication are described and may be a less invasive alternative to open surgery. This review describes the etiology, clinical presentation, diagnosis, and treatment of acquired DP in adults.

ETIOLOGY

The diaphragm is a dome-shaped aponeurotic muscular structure that is enervated by the phrenic nerve, which arises from the third to the fifth cervical nerve roots. From the origin at the level of the scalenus anterior, the phrenic nerve follows a circuitous route in the posterior neck and mediastinum before entering the central tendon of the diaphragm. Because the only enervation of the diaphragm is via the phrenic nerve, total DP can be achieved by compression or damage to the phrenic nerve anywhere along its length (**Fig. 1**). The differential diagnosis of acquired DP is, therefore, broad and includes traumatic, compressive, neurogenic, myopathic, and inflammatory conditions (**Box 1**).

Unilateral DP (UDP) is commonly caused by ipsilateral phrenic nerve palsy. The most common cause of UDP is currently open heart surgery, occurring at an incidence of 2% to 20%.[1,2] The left nerve is more commonly affected than the right, perhaps due to injury during mobilization of the left internal mammary artery.[2] Another theory is that cold cardioplegia induces a direct thermal injury to the phrenic nerve during cardiac arrest.[1,2] In support of this, animal studies have demonstrated that local hypothermia induced by cardioplegia induces acute demyelation and axonal degeneration of the phrenic nerve.[3] In contrast, phrenic nerve injury is relatively uncommon in other noncardiac thoracic surgery, such as lung resections for carcinoma.[4] One exception is during thymectomy for thymoma, where the tumor is often invading or in close proximity to the superior extent of the nerve. The phrenic nerve was intentionally sacrificed for oncologic purposes in approximately 7% of a series of 183 patients.[5] Other rare causes of iatrogenic phrenic nerve palsy include injury after head and neck surgery,[6] chiropractic manipulation,[7] anesthetic blockade,[8] and central venous catheter placement.[9]

Unilateral phrenic nerve palsy can be induced by direct invasion or compression by space-occupying lesions at any point along its length. These include primary neoplasms, most commonly bronchogenic carcinoma or invasive thymoma (see **Box 1**). Less frequently, secondary neoplasms, such as metastatic pulmonary nodules or bulky mediastinal lymphadenopathy, may also lead to unilateral phrenic nerve palsy. Fortunately, most patients with incidentally found UDP do not have an occult intrathoracic

Division of Thoracic Surgery, Department of Surgery, University of Toronto, Toronto General Hospital, 200 Elizabeth Street, Room 9N-955, Toronto, ON, Canada M5G 2C4

* Corresponding author.
E-mail address: Gail.Darling@uhn.on.ca (G.E. Darling).

Thorac Surg Clin 19 (2009) 501–510
doi:10.1016/j.thorsurg.2009.08.011

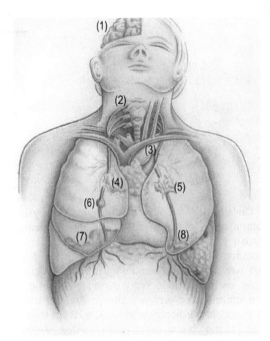

Fig. 1. Etiology of phrenic nerve palsy. DP can be caused by phrenic nerve damage anywhere along its length. (1) ALS. (2) Cervical osteoarthritis. (3) Aortic aneurysm. (4) Thymoma. (5) Lung carcinoma. (6) Peripheral nerve sheath tumor. (7) Pneumonia. (8) Tuberculosis.

malignancy. In a series of 142 patients with incidental diaphragmatic paresis, only 3.5% (n = 5) had an undiagnosed malignancy accounting for their symptoms.[10] Rarely, benign neoplasms, such as intrathoracic goiter[11] or phrenic nerve schwannoma,[12] may also present with unilateral phrenic nerve palsy. Non-neoplastic examples of compressive phrenic neuropathy include cervical osteoarthritis at the C3 to C5 nerve roots,[13] von Recklinghausen's disease,[14] and an expanding aortic aneurysm.[15]

Any peripheral neuropathy may affect the phrenic nerve, causing UDP. These include acute processes, such as MS[16] and chronic inflammatory demyelinating neuropathy.[17] For unknown reasons, diabetic neuropathy has a special predilection for phrenic nerve involvement.[18] Inflammatory conditions may adversely affect phrenic nerve function by causing local injury to the nerve (ie, pneumonia or tuberculosis) or by direct nerve damage, such as in herpes zoster or poliomyelitis.[19] Also, there have been several case reports of radiation therapy causing delayed phrenic nerve palsy several months to years after its administration.[20] If no obvious cause of DP is identified, it is labeled idiopathic. A recent report has suggested that such cases of idiopathic DP may be an acute viral infection of the nerve with herpes zoster; so-called Bell's palsy of the diaphragm.[21] Treatment of these

---

Box 1
Differential diagnosis of acquired diaphragmatic paralysis

1. Traumatic
   a. Penetrating injury
   b. Traction injury
      i. Motor vehicle collision
      ii. Cervical manipulation
   c. Iatrogenic
      i. Head and neck surgery
      ii. Cardiothoracic surgery
      iii. Anesthetic blockade
      iv. Central venous catheter placement

2. External phrenic nerve compression
   a. Neoplastic
      i. Pulmonary tumors
         1. Primary
            a. Non–small cell lung cancer
            b. Small cell lung cancer
            c. Carcinoid
         2. Secondary
      ii. Mediastinal tumors
         1. Thymoma
         2. Lymphoma
         3. Germ cell
         4. Intrathoracic goiter
         5. Phrenic nerve stimulation test
   b. Non-neoplastic
      i. Aortic aneurysm
      ii. von Recklinghausen's disease
      iii. Cervical osteoarthritis

3. Neurogenic
   a. Neuropathy
      i. Multiple sclerosis (MS)
      ii. Chronic inflammatory demyelinating neuropathy
      iii. Diabetic neuropathy
      iv. Amyotrophic lateral sclerosis (ALS)
   b. Brainstem injury
      i. Ischemia
      ii. Compression

4. Inflammatory
   a. Pneumonia
   b. Polio
   c. Inclusion body myositis
   d. Herpes zoster
   e. Vasculitis
   f. Tuberculosis
   g. Radiotherapy

5. Idiopathic

patients with valcyclovir led to symptomatic improvement in this small nonrandomized study.[21]

Bilateral diaphragmatic paralysis (BDP) occurs most often in the context of severe generalized weakness from motor neuron disease or myopathy. Common examples include MS and ALS.[16] Diaphragmatic impairment often parallels the course of the underlying disease but often lags behind clinical improvement of generalized weakness. Other times, the diaphragms are primarily affected without generalized weakness, such as in postpolio syndrome.[22] Myopathies also can cause BDP through direct injury to the muscle itself. Examples include limb-girdle muscle dystrophy, acid malatase deficiency, thyroid disease, and connective tissue disorders.[23] Apart from these causes, the most common cause of BDP is secondary to high spinal cord transection after cervical spine trauma. High cervical spine fracture (C1 to C5) accounts for 37% of all patients who survive acute spinal injury, most commonly in the context of a motor vehicle collision.[24] The degree of impairment of diaphragm function in these cases depends largely on the completeness of injury and the level of transection.

CLINICAL PRESENTATION
Pathophysiology

The diaphragm is the primary muscle of respiration. Diaphragmatic contraction expands intrathoracic volume by displacing the abdominal viscera and lifting/expanding the rib cage using the abdomen as a fulcrum. The resulting negative intrathoracic pressure induces a net influx of air into the lungs. When the diaphragm is paralyzed, work is generated entirely by the accessory muscles of respiration: the intercostals, scalenes, and sternocleidomastoid. When paralyzed, the affected diaphragm remains stationary or, worse, moves paradoxically with respiration. Paradoxic superior movement results in a greatly reduced change in intrathoracic volume with inspiration, leading to a more severe respiratory impairment than if the diaphragm was fixed in position. As the abdominal contents apply pressure on the diaphragms in the supine position, these respiratory derangements are often accentuated when lying flat, a key feature of DP. The clinical presentation of DP is highly variable and depends on the degree of paralysis, the rapidity of onset, whether or not the paralysis is unilateral or bilateral, and the presence of underlying pulmonary disease.

Bilateral Diaphragmatic Paralysis

BDP usually presents with progressive dyspnea that worsens when lying supine. As a result, these patients are often assumed to have congestive heart failure and, therefore, undergo cardiac workup.[25] The orthopnea of BDP is sudden and profound, resulting in severe dyspnea and tachypnea, followed by rapid, shallow breathing. As the diaphragm is the primary muscle of respiration during rapid eye movement sleep, the effects of paralysis are more pronounced at night.[25] Hypoventilation and hypercarbia result, leading to excessive daytime fatigue, anxiety, and morning headaches.[25,26] Chronic hypercarbia can lead to irreversible pulmonary hypertension and cor pulmonale. Patients with BDP are often severely debilitated by their symptoms, with forced expiratory volume in 1 second (FEV_1) values commonly in the range of 45% of predicted or lower.[27,28] Exercise physiology in patients with BDP also reveals significant reductions in endurance and peak minute ventilation.[29] Hypoxemia and secondary erythrocytosis occurs due to alveolar hypoventilation, subsegmental atelectasis, and ventilation-perfusion mismatch. A strong index of suspicion must be maintained for BDP, as the average length of time from onset to diagnosis is 2 years, with a range between 6 weeks to 10 years.[18] In the absence of severe symptoms, the length of the diagnostic delay is significantly longer.[18] In contrast, acute traumatic BDP secondary to high cervical spine injury results in a profound derangement in respiratory mechanics, in most cases leading to severe dyspnea, hypoxia, and need for ventilatory support. In these cases, the diagnosis is obvious.

Unilateral Diaphragmatic Paralysis

UDP is more common than bilateral paralysis, and its presentation is often more subtle. The left diaphragm is more commonly affected than the right and men are more often affected than women.[30] In the absence of intrinsic lung disease, patients are often asymptomatic or have only mild derangements in respiratory mechanics. Accordingly, 50% of all patients are completely asymptomatic and UDP is detected as an incidental finding on a chest radiograph obtained for other reasons.[10] Those who are symptomatic generally describe dyspnea and diminished exercise tolerance on exertion.[10] When formally measured, patients with UDP show significant reductions in exercise endurance and peak minute ventilation compared with normal controls.[29] In a series of 36 patients, there was substantially diminished Pao_2 and breathing capacity in patients with UDP.[30] The condition was not fatal in this cohort.[30] Orthopnea is also seen in UDP as in BDP, although not as pronounced. If intrinsic lung disease is present, symptoms are accentuated and exercise tolerance is more greatly reduced.

DIAGNOSIS
Findings

Physical examination in patients with BDP reveals dramatic onset of dyspnea on assuming the supine position. Careful inspection of the abdominal wall reveals paradoxic upward movement during inspiration, a hallmark of the disease.[31,32] Visible use of the accessory muscles of respiration may be evident, especially if the patients are severely affected. Breath sounds are equally diminished bilaterally, there being no difference between the right and left hemithorax. In contrast, patients with UDP typically have unequal breath sounds with diminished or absent air entry near the base on the affected side. Dullness to percussion and inspiratory crackles may also be present over the paralyzed hemidiaphragm.[32] Dyspnea may also be elicited on assuming the supine position in UDP, although not as pronounced as for BDP.

Pulmonary Function Tests

The role of pulmonary function tests (PFTs) in assessing suspected DP is to (1) confirm the diagnosis, (2) quantify the physiologic effect of DP, and (3) identify the presence of a confounding respiratory disorder. The single most important diagnostic test is a fall in the vital capacity (VC) as measured in the upright and supine positions.[27,33] The normal decrease in VC is less than 10% in healthy subjects, owing to the increase in diaphragmatic tone while lying flat.[27,33] In patients with DP, however, the VC falls in excess of 50% when assuming the supine position, resulting from the cephalad displacement of the abdominal viscera.[27,33] In patients with UDP, the effect is more pronounced in right-sided paralysis, resulting from the weight of the liver.

Patients with UDP and BDP display a restrictive process in upright spirometry. Those with UDP typically demonstrate VC, total lung capacity (TLC), and FEV_1 values of approximately 75%, 85%, and 70% of predicted, respectively.[27,28] Patients with BDP usually have more severe restriction, with VC, TLC, and FEV_1 values of approximately 45%, 55%, and 50%, respectively.[27,28] The functional residual capacity and residual volume is usually unaffected in UDP, whereas atelectasis and compression lower these values by up to 50% of predicted in BDP.[27] The maximal inspiratory pressure is mildly reduced in UDP (70% of predicted) and usually severely diminished in BDP (10%–20% of predicted).[27,28]

PFT should be obtained as a baseline in all cases of diaphragmatic paralysis.

Imaging

In patients with UDP, the diagnosis is strongly suggested by the presence of an elevated hemidiaphragm on the affected side. The other classic features of DP include an accentuated dome configuration in the posteroanterior and lateral projections, with abnormally deepened costophrenic and costovertebral angles.[34] These findings must be interpreted with caution, however, as Chetta and colleagues[35] have found that the true incidence of DP as confirmed by electromyography (EMG) was only 24% of a group of patients referred for an elevated hemidiaphragm. They concluded that the false-negative and false-positive rates of a chest x-ray film were 10% and 56%, respectively, leading to a positive predictive value of only 33%.[35] Therefore, an elevated hemidiaphgram on chest x-ray is a relatively nonspecific finding and confirmatory testing must be done to diagnose UDP.

A frequently cited method of confirmation is the sniff test, wherein diaphragmatic motion during sniffing is recorded using fluoroscopy. Brisk diaphragmatic movement on the normal side and paradoxic elevation of the affected hemidiaphragm are seen in more than 90% of patients who have UDP.[36] Ultrasonography has also been recently described as a novel method of detecting paralysis of the diaphragm.[37,38] Because a normal diaphragm thickens during inspiration whereas a paralyzed diaphragm does not, DP can also be determined by the loss of thickening as seen from functional residual capacity to TLC.[37] M-mode ultrasonography can also directly assess whether or not diaphragmatic movement is absent or paradoxic.[38] Therefore, ultrasonography may be an inexpensive and noninvasive alternative to fluoroscopy, although its interpretation is largely operator dependent. Real-time MRI has also been described, although this method has not gained widespread acceptance.[39]

Although these imaging tests are useful to confirm or exclude the diagnosis in patients with UDP, their utility in BDP is questionable. A plain film is not usually helpful in BDP because both hemidiaphragms are equally affected and only decreased bilateral lung volumes are seen on both sides. Similarly, diaphragmatic movement during a sniff test is often difficult to interpret as there is not a normal hemidiaphragm available for comparison.[36] Often, the paradoxic movement of the diaphragm is masked when the abdominal muscles are recruited to assist in expiration.

Contraction of the rectus muscles during expiration leads to a misleading cranial movement of the diaphragms, thereby mimicking normal respiration. Similarly, passive relaxation of the rectus muscles during inspiration may also result in a normal-appearing caudal movement.[36] Therefore, the fluoroscopic sniff test and its variants are often falsely negative and are not recommended in the confirmation of BDP. Ultrasonographic measurements of diaphragmatic thickness may still be useful in these patients as it is a direct measure of contraction, rather than position.[37]

Electromyography

Measurements of the electrical and mechanical responses to phrenic nerve stimulation can be measured in diaphragmatic EMG.[40–42] Electrical stimulation can be accomplished by using percutaneous needle electrodes in the neck or by single/bilateral magnetic cervical coils.[40–42] Action potentials (APs) are then measured via esophageal electrodes or surface electrodes positioned at the seventh to ninth intercostal spaces. The mechanical response is measured by the change in trans-diaphragmatic pressure (Pdi) determined by the pressure differential between the esophagus (pleural pressure) and the stomach (abdominal pressure). Most neuropathic conditions demonstrate increased latency times with markedly diminished or absent APs.[40,41] Phrenic nerve injury or compression may also show a similar pattern, whereas transection is usually demonstrated by a complete absence of APs.[40] In contrast, myopathic conditions do not display impairment of nerve conduction or propagation but show markedly diminished Pdi.[40,41] Tidal breathing, sniff Pdi, and Pdimax (maximal inspiratory effort against a closed glottis) are effort dependent, subject to variability, and thus unreliable in the diagnosis of DP.[42] Therefore, the stimulated twitch or titanic Pdi is recommended to standardize against variability in patient effort.[42] As with all EMG studies, specialized expertise is required for their measurement and interpretation. They remain, however, the gold standard in the diagnosis of DP.

MANAGEMENT

Because treatments of BDP and UDP are different, they are treated separately.

Unilateral Diaphragmatic Paralysis

Once a diagnosis of UDP is confirmed, every effort should be made to exclude major intrathoracic pathology, such as active infection, inflammation, or malignancy, that requires urgent treatment. Contrast-enhanced, high-resolution thoracic CT scan is usually sufficient in this regard. Once this is addressed, a careful history regarding the extent of respiratory limitation should be obtained and the presence of any confounding respiratory disease. Onset, timing, and severity of respiratory symptoms and the impact such symptoms have on a patient's lifestyle should be ascertained. Supine and upright PFT should be obtained as a baseline and any confirmatory tests if the diagnosis is in doubt. In the absence of other respiratory illness, most patients with UDP tolerate hemi-DP well, with only 25% of patients having symptoms.[10] If the injury is minor, phrenic nerve recovery can often be observed provided that there is no underlying neuropathic process.[43] Patients with stable respiratory function who are asymptomatic or mildly symptomatic can, therefore, be safely observed.

Surgery for idiopathic UDP remains controversial due to the rarity of the disease and the relatively benign natural course of the illness. Indications for surgery include (1) lifestyle-modifying dyspnea or orthopnea, (2) evidence of severe impairment on upright and supine PFTs, and (3) progression or nonresolution of symptomatology. Surgical correction of UDP involves diaphragmatic plication, whereby the diaphragm is sutured to become a fixed, immobile structure. This transfixion eliminates the paradoxic movement of the diaphragm with inspiration, thereby improving the ability of the accessory muscles to create a negative inspiratory pressure. The diaphragm may be indicated through a standard posterolateral thoracotomy incision in the eighth intercostal space or by laparoscopy or thoracoscopy. A series of six to eight nonabsorbable U-shaped sutures are then placed with care in the attenuated diaphragm, with care not to damage underlying abdominal viscera (Fig. 2). Redundant tissue can then be covered closed using interrupted sutures. The final result is a taut, immobile diaphragm that is not drawn into the chest during inspiration (see Fig. 2).

Several studies have analyzed the short- and long-term results of diaphragmatic plication in symptomatic patients with UDP. In 1990, Graham and colleagues[44] reported a series of 17 patients who underwent open thoracotomy and diaphragmatic plication for idiopathic UDP. All patients had moderate hypoxemia that improved significantly following plication; these results were durable after 5-year follow-up. This study was hampered, however, by incomplete follow-up in 11 of 17 patients. Higgs and colleagues[45] reported on their series of 19 patients with plication for

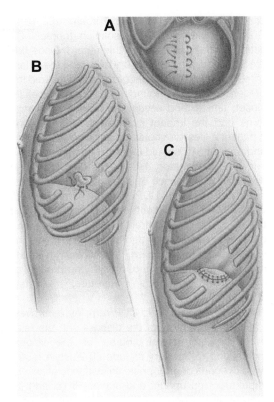

Fig. 2. Technique of diaphragm plication. (*A*) Plication is performed with six to eight nonabsorbable U-shaped stitches placed in the diaphgram. (*B*) Diaphragm is taut and immobile after sutures are tied. (*C*) Redundant tissue is imbricated.

symptomatic UDP with a mean follow-up of 10 years (range 7–14). All of the patients in this series had severe lifestyle limiting symptomatology and many were unable to work. The mean preoperative FEV_1, forced vital capacity (FVC), and TLC were 71%, 67%, and 74%, respectively, of predicted in this cohort of patients.[45] These patients experienced significant improvements in supine and upright spirometry at 6-week follow-up, with a mean postoperative FEV_1, FVC, and TLC of 81.1%, 79.8%, and 83.2%, respectively, of predicted (all values, $P<0.001$).[45] These results were durable at 5-year follow-up, with significant long-term improvement in these spirometry parameters.[45] Furthermore, 12 of 19 patients demonstrated improvement in Medical Research Council (MRC) and American Thoracic Society dyspnea scales of greater than 1 point, with only one patient with stable symptoms and two with worsening dyspnea.[45] Although encouraging, this study was limited by the lack of a control group. Therefore, the effects of surgery cannot be ascertained based on the known benign natural history of the disease.

The largest series of open diaphragmatic plication was reported by Versteegh and colleagues[46] on a series of 22 consecutive patients with a mean follow-up of 4.9 years. In this report, symptomatic patients with fluoroscopically verified DP were offered open thoracotomy and diaphragm plication. All patients in this series had severe dyspnea in the supine position, with three patients requiring CPAP ventilation at night and two patients with pulmonary hypertension. Five patients in this series had BDP and underwent bilateral staged thoracotomy for diaphragm plication. Pre- and postoperative spirometry were performed and quality of life was assessed by the transition dyspnea index score. Patients experienced a statistically significant improvement of FEV_1 and VC at long-term follow-up (64% versus 71% and 70% vs 79%, $P<0.03$).[46] The benefits were even more pronounced in the supine position (FEV_1 45% vs 63%, $P>0.02$; VC 54% vs 73%, $P<0.03$).[46] There was a trend to a larger magnitude of benefit from diaphragmatic plication in patients with worse preoperative spirometry results.[46] Mean postoperative improvement in transition dyspnea index score was +5.69, which represents a substantial improvement.[46] Furthermore, all patients were able to sleep in the supine position postoperatively with all three patients weaned off of nighttime CPAP. There were three in-hospital deaths in this series accounting for 13% of the total series.[46] One patient died of myocardial infarction, one of pulmonary embolus, and another from right heart failure from pulmonary hypertension.[46] Furthermore, four patients complained of chronic post-thoracotomy pain syndrome in follow-up. This series illustrates that diaphragmatic plication is not a trivial operation and has a substantial risk for morbidity and mortality.

Due to the morbidity of open thoracotomy, Freeman and colleagues[47] reported on a series of 25 patients undergoing diaphragmatic plication for UDP, 22 of whom had thoracoscopic repair. In this nonrandomized study, 33 patients met the inclusion criteria of having lifestyle-limiting dyspnea (MRC dyspnea scale 3 or more) and fluoroscopically proved UDP. Of these, 25 agreed to plication and seven patients declined. All patients received aggressive pulmonary rehabilitation under the supervision of a respirologist.[47] Conversion to open operation occurred in three patients, all of whom had a body mass index greater than 30.[47] The mean length of stay was shorter in the thoracoscopy group compared to the open group (3.7 versus 5.4 days).[47] Patients who underwent plication had significant improvements in FEV_1 (+21.4%), TLC (+16.1%), and FRV (+20%) at 6 months' follow-up.[47] Mean improvement in MRC scores was 1.9, with most patients becoming only mildly symptomatic in the postoperative period. In contrast, the seven patients who declined operative plication experienced no significant change in their mean spirometry or MRC scores at the 6-months' follow-up. These patients also had an average of 1.3 hospital admissions for dyspnea in the intervening time period.[46] The investigators conclude that video-assisted diaphragmatic plication is a safe and effective procedure in relieving symptoms in patients with UDP. Furthermore, the nonoperative group demonstrated no such improvement in this nonrandomized study even with best medical management and aggressive pulmonary rehabilitation.[46] The major limitation of this study is the short (6 month) follow-up. Further study is needed to determine if these changes are durable.

Groth and colleagues[48] has recently reported on a series of 22 patients who underwent laparoscopic diaphragmatic plication at the 2009 annual meeting for the American Association for Thoracic Surgery. The laparoscopic approach is potentially beneficial due to the absence of a chest incision, potentially faster recovery, and the placement of redundant tissue within the abdomen, obviating imbricating this tissue at the time of plication. The potential drawbacks are the generation of a sympathetic pleural effusion that requires drainage and the inability to perform the procedure on the right-hand side, owing to the presence of the liver on this side. Similar to the thoracoscopic repair, preliminary results demonstrate significantly improved percent predicted forced vital capacity (FVC %), FEV_1, and forced inspiratory flow rate, which are durable to at least 12 months.[48] The ability to perform a minimally invasive repair through the abdomen is a novel method to avoid the potential complications of thoracotomy for this disease.

Summary

Drawing on the available evidence from these small single-institution case series, diaphragmatic plication is indicated for symptomatic relief of dyspnea from UDP. The open series have demonstrated substantial and durable improvements in spirometry and dyspnea scales, although at a not insignificant risk of morbidity and mortality. The lone thoracoscopic series confirms the remarkable improvement in symptom scales and objective testing seen in open thoracotomy, with perhaps lower morbidity and mortality. Ideally a randomized trial would substantiate these conclusions, however, due to the rarity of the disease, a RCT may be impossible to complete.

Bilateral Diaphragmatic Paralysis

The majority of patients with BDP present with steadily progressive dyspnea that necessitates some form of treatment. Once the diagnosis is established, aggressive respiratory support is indicated because the majority of patients with mild to moderate BDP achieve significant symptomatic improvement with noninvasive ventilation.[49–52] This suggests that the pathogenesis of respiratory failure in these patients is primarily due to fatigue of the accessory muscles of respiration. In the initial report by Davis and colleagues,[49] a negative pressure cuirass respirator improved the hypercapnic respiratory failure in a series of patients with BDP. This benefit has been replicated in other forms of negative pressure ventilatory support[51] and in the modern use of positive pressure support, such as CPAP.[52] The beneficial effects of these devices are most pronounced during rapid eye movement sleep, in which the diaphragm is usually the primary muscle of respiration.[25] Nighttime CPAP or negative pressure support is usually enough to improve or reverse the hypoxic and hypercapnic respiratory failure seen on arterial blood gas analysis in patients with BDP.[49–52] In the modern era, CPAP is usually the support method of first choice, with older methods of negative pressure support (such as cuirass, rocking bed, or plume-wrap) reserved for those who cannot tolerate nasal or oral positive pressure ventilation.[52] The use of negative pressure ventilation must be used with caution as it may exacerbate upper airway obstruction in patients with obstructive sleep apnea. Dedicated sleep studies are, therefore, recommended for those patients in whom negative pressure ventilation is considered.[50]

Those patients with severe BDP or those with concomitant pulmonary disease who cannot maintain ventilation by any other means are candidates for permanent tracheostomy and mechanical ventilation, as are patients with life-threatening illness or sudden and complete loss of bilateral diaphragm function, such as those with high spinal cord injury. The prognosis of these patients is usually poor, as might be expected from the severity of the underlying problem and the constellation of complications related to chronic mechanical ventilatory support.

Although diaphragmatic plication has been described in BDP,[46] it must be used with caution, as many causes of phrenic nerve palsy are reversible and spontaneous recovery of a plicated diaphragm may actually impair ventilation.[43] If surgery for BDP is considered, an adequate time period to allow spontaneous recovery of diaphragm function must have elapsed, and clear evidence of paradoxic motion by fluoroscopy should be documented.

DIAPHRAGM PACING

Diaphragmatic pacing is a method to stimulate contraction in select patients with UDP or BDP.[53] Pacing can be accomplished by electrical stimulation of the phrenic nerve or by direct stimulation of the muscle itself. In order for phrenic nerve pacing to be successful, the nerve must be intact and there should be no diffuse myopathy.[53] An ideal patient is someone with a high cervical spine injury (C1/C2) who is otherwise ventilator dependent. Patients with C3, C4, or C5 injuries are not candidates for this procedure as the phrenic nerve cell bodies are damaged by the fracture/transection. Pacing is also not possible if the nerve is transected, because without proximal stimulation the nerve atrophies, rendering it incapable of stimulation.[54] This problem can be circumvented by autologous nerve transposition via end-end anastomosis from the fourth intercostal to the phrenic nerve.[54] Axonal regeneration and successful diaphragmatic pacing was achieved in 8 of 10 patients with midcervical spine fractures.[54]

Electrical stimulation of the phrenic nerve can be achieved by electrodes placed in the chest or in the neck.[53,55] Placement in the neck avoids a thoracotomy but can result in undesirable upper extremity twitching via stimulation of the brachial plexus. Glenn and colleagues[53] reported his experience with this technique and found that 46% of patients with bilateral diaphragmatic pacing became respirator-free.[55] Another single institution series reviewed their long-term results from phrenic nerve pacing in 22 patients.[56] All but two patients were successfully paced with 22% of patients paced for 10 years or more.[56] The frequency and amplitude of pacing must be carefully monitored, however, lest irreversible muscular damage occur.[55] This technique should, therefore, only be carried out in high-volume centers with specialized experience in the technique.

Direct pacing of the diaphragm muscle may also be carried out via electrodes implanted directly into the muscle via laparoscopy.[57] Onders and colleagues[57] described a series of five patients who underwent this procedure, with three of them using pacing as their sole means of ventilatory support. Until more experience is generated with this technique, however, it should be considered to be experimental.

SUMMARY

Acquired DP in adults is multifactorial. Symptoms largely depend on whether or not the paresis is unilateral or bilateral and on the etiology, onset, progression, and presence of underlying pulmonary disease. UDP is a well-tolerated condition with a favorable prognosis. Diaphragmatic plication is indicated in carefully selected patients with UDP and can be done by minimally invasive techniques. Patients with BDP are usually severely symptomatic and require some form of mechanical ventilatory support. Diaphragmatic pacing is an option for a select group of patients with BDP in centers with specialized expertise.

ACKNOWLEDGEMENTS

We are indebted to Cheryl Vollings for her excellent artwork for the figures.

REFERENCES

1. Dimopoulou I, Daganou M, Dafni U, et al. Phrenic nerve dysfunction after cardiac operations: electrophysiologic evaluation of risk factors. Chest 1998; 113:8–14.
2. Olopade CO, Staats BA. Time course of recovery from frostbitten phrenics after coronary artery bypass graft surgery. Chest 1991;99:1112–5.
3. Marco JD, Hahn JW, Barner HB. Topical cardiac hypothermia and phrenic nerve injury. Ann Thorac Surg 1977;23:235–7.
4. De Troyer A, Vanderhoeft P. Phrenic nerve function after pneumonectomy. Chest 1982;81:212–4.
5. Salati M, Cardillo G, Carbone L, et al. Iatrogenic phrenic nerve injury durning thymectomy: the extent of the problem. J. Thorac Cardiovasc Surg 2009, in press.
6. Yaddanapudi S, Shah SC. Bilateral phrenic nerve injury after neck dissection: an uncommon cause of respiratory failure. J Laryngol Otol 1996;110: 281–3.
7. Schram DJ, Vosik W, Cantral D. Diaphragmatic paralysis following cervical chiropractic manipulation: case report and review. Chest 2001;119(2): 638–40.
8. Erickson JM, Louis SD, Naughton NN. Symptomatic phrenic nerve palsy after supraclavicular block in an obese man. Orthopedics 2009;32:368.
9. Takasaki Y, Arai T. Transient right phrenic nerve palsy associated with central venous catheterization. Br J Anaesth 2001;87(3):510–1.
10. Piehler JM, Pairolero PC, Gracey DR, et al. Unexplained diaphragmatic paralysis: a harbinger of malignant disease? J Thorac Cardiovasc Surg 1982;84:861–4.

11. Van Doorn LG, Kranendonk SE. Partial unilateral phrenic nerve paralysis caused by a large intrathoracic goiter. Neth J Med 1996;48(6):216–9.

12. Mevio E, Gorini E, Sbrocca M, et al. Unusual cases of cervical nerves schwannomas: phrenic and vagus nerve involvement. Auris Nasus Larynx 2003; 30(2):209–13.

13. Mellem H, Johansen B, Nakstad P, et al. Unilateral phrenic nerve paralysis caused by osteoarthritis of the cervical spine. Eur J Respir Dis 1987;71:56–8.

14. Hassoun PM, Celli BR. Bilateral diaphragm paralysis secondary to central von Recklinghausen's disease. Chest 2000;117:1196–200.

15. Rabago G, Martin-Trenor A, Lopez-Coronado JL. Chronic aneurysm of the descending thoracic aorta: presenting with right pleural effusion and left phrenic nerve palsy. Tex Heart Inst J 1999;26(1):96–8.

16. Balbierz JM, Ellenberg M, Honet JC. Complete hemidiaphragmatic paralysis in a patient with multiple sclerosis. Am J Phys Med Rehabil 1988;67:161–5.

17. Stojkovic T, De Seze J, Hurtevent JF, et al. Phrenic nerve palsy as a feature of chronic inflammatory demyelinating polyradiculoneuropathy. Muscle Nerve 2003;27:497–9.

18. Chan CK, Loke J, Virgulto JA, et al. Bilateral diaphragmatic paralysis: clinical spectrum, prognosis, and diagnostic approach. Arch Phys Med Rehabil 1988;67:161–5.

19. Stowasser M, Cameron J, Oliver WA. Diaphragmatic paralysis following cervical herpes zoster. Med J Aust 1990;153:555–6.

20. Brander PE, Jarvinen V, Lohela P, et al. Bilateral diaphragmatic weakness: a late complication of radiotherapy. Thorax 1997;52:829–31.

21. Crausman RS, Summerhill EM, McCool FD. Idiopathic diaphragmatic paralysis: Bell's palsy of the diaphragm? Lung 2009;187:153–7.

22. Imai T, Matsumoto H. Insidious phrenic nerve involvement in postpolio syndrome. Intern Med 2006;45(8):563–4.

23. Aldrich TK, Aldrich MS. Primary muscle diseases: respiratory mechanisms and complications. In: Kamholz SL, editor. Pulmonary aspects of neurologic disease. New York: SP Scientific and Medical Books; 1986. p. 85–110.

24. Cripps RA. Spinal cord injury, Australia 2004–5. Injury research and statistics series number 29. 2006. Adelaide (SA): AIHW; (AIHW cat no. INJCAT 86).

25. Skatrud J, Iber C, McHugh W, et al. Determinants of hypoventilation during wakefulness and sleep in diaphragmatic paralysis. Am Rev Respir Dis 1980;121: 587–93.

26. Sajkov D, Marshall R, Walker P, et al. Sleep apnoea related hypoxia is associated with cognitive disturbances in patients with tetraplegia. Spinal Cord 1998;36:231–9.

27. Allen SM, Hunt B, Green M. Fall in vital capacity with posture. Br J Dis Chest 1985;79:267–71.

28. Fromageot C, Lofaso F, Annane D, et al. Supine fall in lung volumes in the assessment of diaphragmatic weakness in neuromuscular disorders. Arch Phys Med Rehabil 2001;82:123–8.

29. Hart N, Nickol AH, Cramer D, et al. Effect of severe isolated unilateral and bilateral diaphragm weakness on exercise performance. Am J Respir Crit Care Med 2002;165:1265.

30. Elefteriades J, Singh M, Tang P, et al. Unilateral diaphragm paralysis: etiology, impact and natural history. J Cardiovas surg (Torino) 2008;49:289–95.

31. Incalzi RA, Capparella O, Gemma A, et al. Diaphragmatic paralysis: a difficult diagnosis. Postgrad Med J 1990;66:880.

32. Ben-Dov I, Kaminski N, Reichert N, et al. Diaphragmatic paralysis: a clinical imitator of cardiorespiratory diseases. Isr Med Assoc J 2008;10:579–83.

33. Mier-Jedrzejowicz A, Brophy C, Moxham J, et al. Assessment of diaphragm weakness. Am Rev Respir Dis 1988;137:877.

34. Fraser RS, Muller NL, Colman N, et al. The diaphragm. In: Fraser RS, editor. Diagnosis of disease of the chest. vol. 4. Philadelphia: WB Saunders Company; 1999. p. 2987–3010.

35. Chetta A, Rehman A, Moxham J, et al. Chest radiography cannot predict diaphragm function. Respir Med 2005;99:39–44.

36. Alexander C. Diaphragm movements and the diagnosis of diaphragmatic paralysis. Clin Radiol 1966; 17:79.

37. Gottesman E, McCool FD. Ultrasound evaluation of the paralyzed diaphragm. Am J Respir Crit Care Med 1997;155(5):1570–4.

38. Lloyd T, Tang YM, Benson MD, et al. Diaphragmatic paralysis: the use of M mode ultrasound for diagnosis in adults. Spinal Cord 2006;44(8):505–8.

39. Taylor AM, Jhooti P, Keegan J, et al. Magnetic resonance navigator echo diaphragm monitoring in patients with suspected diaphragm paralysis. J Magn Reson Imaging 1999;9:69–74.

40. Moxham J, Grassino A. ATS/ERS statement on respiratory muscle testing. Am J Respir Crit Care Med 2002;166:518–624.

41. Kumar N, Folger WN, Bolton CF. Dyspnea as the predominant manifestation of bilateral phrenic neuropathy. Mayo Clin Proc 2004;79:1563.

42. Ciccolella DE, Daly BD, Celli BR. Improved diaphragmatic function after surgical placation for unilateral diaphragmatic paralysis. Am Rev Respir Dis 1992;146:797.

43. Dernaika TA, Younis WG, Carlile PV. Spontaneous recovery in idiopathic unilateral diaphragmatic paralysis. Respir Care 2008;53:341–54.

44. Graham DR, Kaplan D, Evans CC, et al. Diaphragmatic plication for unilateral diaphragmatic

paralysis: a 10-year experience. Ann Thorac Surg 1990;49:248–51.

45. Higgs SM, Hussain A, Jackson M, et al. Long term results of diaphragmatic plication for unilateral diaphragm paralysis. Eur J Cardiothorac Surg 2002; 21:294–7.

46. Versteegh M, Braun J, Voigt PG, et al. Diaphragm plication in adult patients with diaphragm paralysis leads to long-term improvement of pulmonary function and level of dyspnea. Eur J Cardiothorac Surg 2007;32:449–56.

47. Freeman RK, Wozniak TC, Fitzgerald EB. Functional and physiologic results of video-assisted thoracoscopic diaphragm plication in adult patients with unilateral diaphragm paralysis. Ann Thorac Surg 2006;81:1853–7.

48. Groth SS, Rueth NM, Klopp A. Laparoscopic diaphragm plication: an objective evaluation of short and mid term results. AATS 2009 published abstract.

49. Davis J, Goldman M, Loh L, et al. Diaphragm function and alveolar hypoventilation. Q J Med 1976;45:87.

50. Gibson GJ. Diaphragmatic paresis: pathophysiology, clinical features and investigation. Thorax 1989;44:960.

51. Celli B, Rassulo J, Caral R. Ventilatory muscle dysfunction in patients with bilateral idiopathic diaphragmatic paralysis; reversal by intermittent external negative pressure ventilation. Am Rev Respir Dis 1987;136:1276.

52. Hill N. Non-invasive ventilation. Am Rev Respir Dis 1994;147:1050.

53. Glenn WW. The treatment of respiratory paralysis by diaphragm pacing. Ann Thorac Surg 1980;30: 106.

54. Kriger LM, Krieger AJ. The intercostal to phrenic nerve transfer: an effective means of reanimation g the diaphragm in patients with high cervical spine injury. Plast Reconstr Surg 2000;105:1255–61.

55. Glen WW, Hogan JF, Loke JS, et al. Ventilatory support by pacing of the conditioned diaphragm in quadriplegia. N Engl J Med 1984;310:1150.

56. Garrido-Garcia H, Mazaira A, Martin E, et al. Treatment of chronic ventilatory failure using a diaphragmatic pacemaker. Spinal Cord 1998;36:310.

57. Onders RP, Dimarco AF, Ignagni AR, et al. Mapping the phrenic nerve motor point: the key to a successful laparoscopic diaphragm pacing system in the first human series. Surgery 2004;136:819–26.

Diaphragmatic Eventration

Shawn S. Groth, MD[a], Rafael S. Andrade, MD[b],*

KEYWORDS

- Diaphragmatic eventration • Diaphragm plication
- Diaphragmatic paralysis • Laparoscopy • Quality of life

Diaphragmatic eventration is an uncommon condition that is usually discovered incidentally in patients who are asymptomatic and who have an elevated hemidiaphragm on chest X ray. The etiology and pathology of diaphragmatic eventration and paralysis are distinct; however, the clinical presentation in adults is similar and these two conditions are sometimes impossible to distinguish from each other. The treatment for symptomatic patients with diaphragmatic eventration and paralysis is the same: diaphragm plication. Minimally invasive diaphragm plication techniques are now effective alternatives to open plication. This review focuses on the etiology, pathophysiology, diagnosis, and treatment of diaphragmatic eventration in adults.

ETIOLOGY

True diaphragmatic eventration is a congenital developmental defect in the muscular portion of the diaphragm with preserved attachments to the sternum, ribs, and dorsolumbar spine.[1] Diaphragmatic eventration is rare (incidence <0.05%), is more common in males, and more often affects the left hemidiaphragm.[2–4] Embryologic theory postulates that abnormal or delayed migration of myoblasts from the upper cervical somites leads to a structural deficiency of diaphragmatic muscle.[5–7]

In contrast to true diaphragmatic eventration, diaphragmatic paresis or paralysis is a more common, acquired condition that generally results from tumor- or trauma-related phrenic nerve injury.[8–13]

PATHOLOGY

Diaphragmatic eventration can be bilateral, unilateral, total, and localized (anterior, posterolateral, and medial)[6]; localized eventrations can affect any portion of the diaphragm.[1] Microscopically, the eventrated portion has diffuse fibroelastic changes and a paucity of muscle fibers.[14,15] Patients who have diaphragmatic paralysis have a normal amount of muscle fibers, albeit atrophic.

PATHOPHYSIOLOGY AND CLINICAL PRESENTATION

Most adult patients who have diaphragmatic eventration are asymptomatic and generally present with an elevated hemidiaphragm discovered incidentally on a chest X ray.[2,7] Some patients who have diaphragmatic eventration do not become symptomatic until adulthood because of weight gain or because of a change in lung or chest-wall compliance.[7]

Dyspnea on exertion and orthopnea (because of further cranial displacement of the affected hemidiaphragm when supine) are the main symptoms of an elevated hemidiaphragm. Normal caudal movement of the diaphragm during inspiration increases thoracic volume and is pivotal for appropriate lung inflation. Patients who have diaphragmatic eventration may not have the normal caudal movement of the diaphragm necessary for appropriate inspiration[16]; diaphragmatic movement can be diminished, absent, or even paradoxic. As a result, ventilation and perfusion to the basal portion of the lung ipsilateral to the

[a] Department of Surgery, University of Minnesota, MMC 207, 420 Delaware Street, SE, Minneapolis, MN 55455, USA
[b] Division of General Thoracic and Foregut Surgery, Department of Surgery, University of Minnesota, MMC 207, 420 Delaware Street, SE, Minneapolis, MN 55455, USA
* Corresponding author.
E-mail address: andr0119@umn.edu (R.S. Andrade).

Thorac Surg Clin 19 (2009) 511–519
doi:10.1016/j.thorsurg.2009.08.003
1547-4127/09/$ – see front matter © 2009 Elsevier Inc. All rights reserved.

eventrated diaphragm are impaired[17]; ventilation/perfusion mismatch and loss of chest-wall compliance are among the factors that contribute to dyspnea. Some patients develop mild hypoxemia and attempt to compensate by hyperventilating, which can result in mild respiratory alkalosis.[4,18] Other patients (especially those with left hemidiaphragm eventration) can develop nonspecific gastrointestinal symptoms, such as epigastric pain, bloating, heartburn, regurgitation, belching, nausea, constipation, and inability to gain weight.[6,7]

DIAGNOSIS

The evaluation of patients who are symptomatic and who have diaphragmatic eventration should include an objective assessment of dyspnea, physical examination, pulmonary function tests, and imaging studies. The diagnosis of symptomatic hemidiaphragm eventration is primarily clinical, and relies mostly on history, chest X ray, and the physician's clinical acuity.

Symptom Evaluation

A careful history of the duration and progression of dyspnea and orthopnea is critical. Patients who have diaphragm paralysis can often recall when dyspnea started or worsened (eg, after cardiac surgery); patients who have eventration may not be able to determine a specific starting point. Clearly, any additional causes for dyspnea (eg, morbid obesity, primary lung disease, heart failure, and so forth) should be investigated and corrected if possible, because dyspnea secondary to diaphragmatic eventration or paralysis is mainly a diagnosis of exclusion.

All patients who have dyspnea secondary to diaphragmatic eventration should fill out a standardized respiratory questionnaire to evaluate the severity of their symptoms and to assess the response to treatment.

Physical Examination

Physical examination adds little to the diagnosis of diaphragmatic eventration. Nonetheless, two characteristic findings may be present and are worth mentioning: (1) paradoxic inward movement of the lower costal margin during inspiration (known as Hoover's sign),[19] and (2) abdominal paradox (the rib cage and abdomen move out of phase with each other).[16,20] Other nonspecific respiratory signs include diminished maximal excursion of the diaphragm on percussion, diminished breath sounds, and increased anteroposterior diameter of the chest.[6,16] If an eventrated

diaphragm is exceptionally redundant, a flopping sound may be heard on auscultation.[21]

Pulmonary Function Tests

Pulmonary function tests (PFT) may provide an objective measure useful in the assessment of patients who are dyspneic and who have an elevated hemidiaphragm. Because diaphragm dysfunction reduces the compliance of the chest wall, a restrictive pattern (ie, low forced vital capacity [FVC] and forced expiratory volume in 1 second [FEV_1]) is often seen.[4]

The diaphragm is a critical mediator of inspiration; therefore, assessing inspiratory PFT parameters (eg, maximum forced inspiratory flow [FIFmax]) is important.

Additionally, FVC should be assessed in the upright and supine position. Supine FVC in healthy individuals can decrease up to 20% from upright values,[22] and supine lung volumes may decrease by 20% to 50% in patients who have diaphragmatic eventration or paralysis.[18,23,24]

Although PFT are often abnormal in symptomatic patients who have diaphragmatic eventration, these changes are neither consistent nor do they correlate with the severity of dyspnea. The main value of PFT is to provide an objective evaluation of the result of surgery.

Imaging Studies

Chest X ray

On a standard full-inspiration posteroanterior and lateral (PA/LAT) chest X ray, the right hemidiaphragm is normally 1 to 2 cm higher than the left.[25] Hemidiaphragm elevation can be a sign of diaphragmatic eventration or paralysis; however, this is a nonspecific finding because a variety of pulmonary (ie, atelectasis and fibrosis), pleural (ie, pleural effusions and masses), and subdiaphragmatic processes (ie, hepatomegaly, splenomegaly, gastric dilatation, and subphrenic abscesses) can also cause elevation of a hemidiaphragm.[26] Consequently, further studies may be needed if an elevated hemidiaphragm is noted on a chest X ray in the presence of dyspnea.

Fluoroscopic sniff test

During fluoroscopy, patients are instructed to sniff, and diaphragmatic excursion is assessed. Normally, the diaphragm moves caudally. In patients who have hemidiaphragmatic paralysis, the diaphragm may (paradoxically) move cranially. Patients who have diaphragmatic eventration, however, may also exhibit passive upward movement of the diaphragm when sniffing.[6]

Fluoroscopy findings should be interpreted with caution. First, approximately 6% of normal individuals exhibit paradoxic motion on fluoroscopy[27]; to increase the specificity of this study, at least 2 cm of paradoxic motion should be noticed.[16] Second, an eventrated or paralyzed hemidiaphragm may move very little or not at all, without paradoxic motion, making the interpretation of the sniff test and the distinction between paralysis and eventration even more challenging.

Ultrasound

Ultrasound (US) can be used to assess the thickness and the change of thickness of the diaphragm during respiration; it has approximately 80% concordance with fluoroscopy findings.[26–30] However, US has not been validated in clinical practice.

CT

The principal utility of CT scans is to exclude the presence of a cervical or intrathoracic tumor as the cause of phrenic nerve paralysis or to evaluate the possibility of a subphrenic process as the cause of hemidiaphragm elevation. However, a CT scan is not routinely required if the clinical suspicion of an alternate process is low.

MRI

Dynamic MRI can be used to assess diaphragmatic motion.[31] As compared with fluoroscopy, which can assess only motion of the highest points of the diaphragm, it has the advantage of enabling the study of the motion of segments of the diaphragm in multiple planes.[26] However, MRI is more expensive, more time consuming, more uncomfortable for patients than fluoroscopy, and the additional information on segmental diaphragmatic motion is of no clinical value. Consequently, the authors do not recommend MRI as a routine tool for the evaluation of patients who are symptomatic with hemidiaphragm elevation.

Functional Studies

Maximal transdiaphragmatic pressure

The maximal transdiaphragmatic pressure (Pdimax) serves as a surrogate for the force generated by the diaphragm. To measure Pdimax (the difference between intra-abdominal and intrathoracic pressures), pressure transducers are placed inside the stomach (to approximate intra-abdominal pressure) and the esophagus (to approximate intrathoracic pressure[32]). However, this technique is not commonly used to assess patients who have diaphragmatic dysfunction because (1) it is inconvenient, (2) the choice of methodology significantly impacts the Pdimax and reproducibility of the

results,[33] (3) there is a lack of consensus on the most appropriate procedural technique,[33,34] (4) there are no population-based norms,[32] (5) there can be significant intra- and interindividual variability,[26,32] and (6) it is not critical in aiding the clinician to decide whether diaphragm elevation is responsible for dyspnea.

Phrenic nerve conduction studies

Phrenic nerve function can be assessed by stimulating the nerve transcutaneously in the neck.[16,32] In addition to assessing conduction time (normal, < 9.5 milliseconds),[35] phrenic nerve conduction studies can be coupled with (1) diaphragmatic electromyography using surface electrodes to measure the action potential of the diaphragm[35] or (2) Pdimax assessment during phrenic nerve stimulation.[36] This test is of little clinical value since it is cumbersome and is not essential to determine whether dyspnea is secondary to hemidiaphragm elevation.

In summary, to establish that diaphragmatic eventration or paralysis is clinically relevant, patients must have dyspnea that cannot be solely attributed to another process (ie, primary lung or heart disease) and must have an elevated hemidiaphragm on a PA/LAT chest X ray. On occasion it is impossible to clinically differentiate eventration from paralysis; however, this distinction is not essential, as long as the physician establishes that hemidiaphragm elevation is the main cause for dyspnea and that a potentially serious cause for paralysis (ie, tumor or neuromuscular disorder) is not overlooked. A sniff test demonstrating paradoxic motion adds to the evidence that dyspnea is secondary to diaphragm paralysis (or on occasion eventration), but a negative sniff test does not exclude hemidiaphragm elevation as the main cause of dyspnea. PFT are of value in objectively assessing patients' response to diaphragmatic plication. The authors evaluate all patients who have symptomatic hemidiaphragm elevation, whether eventration or paralysis, with a standardized respiratory questionnaire, a PA/LAT chest X ray, and PFT; the authors obtain a sniff test only if they cannot clearly ascertain that dyspnea is secondary to diaphragm dysfunction.

TREATMENT: DIAPHRAGMATIC PLICATION

Surgical repair of diaphragmatic eventration was first described in 1923.[37] Since then, a variety of open and minimally invasive diaphragm plication techniques have been described to reduce symptomatic dysfunctional diaphragm excursion during respiration. Diaphragmatic pacing is an option generally reserved for patients who are quadriplegic and have bilateral diaphragmatic paralysis,[38–40] and has not been established as a practical approach to unilateral diaphragm eventration or paralysis. This section reviews diaphragm plication for unilateral hemidiaphragm eventration with particular emphasis on laparoscopic diaphragm plication.

Operative Indications

The only goal of diaphragm plication is to treat dyspnea; hence, operative intervention is indicated exclusively for patients who are symptomatic. An elevated hemidiaphragm or paradoxic motion per se does not warrant surgery in the absence of significant dyspnea. For adults who have phrenic nerve injury from cardiac surgery, a 1- to 2-year period of observation is often recommended since phrenic nerve function may improve with time[9,10,30,41]; however, patients who are severely symptomatic may warrant a minimally invasive plication even after 6 months, because dyspnea from diaphragm paralysis can significantly impact quality of life and rehabilitation.

Relative contraindications to diaphragm plication are morbid obesity and certain neuromuscular disorders. Ideally, patients who are morbidly obese should be evaluated for medical or surgical bariatric treatment before plication, because dyspnea may improve after significant weight loss and a plication may no longer be warranted. Any type of plication is challenging in patients who are morbidly obese; the degree of plication may be compromised because of technical difficulties, the relief of dyspnea may be limited, and complications are likely. Patients who have neuromuscular disorders, such as amyotrophic lateral sclerosis or muscular dystrophy, should be approached with extreme caution. The benefits of plication on dyspnea are moderate at best, and complications are common. An individualized multidisciplinary approach is necessary to decide on a plication in patients who have morbid obesity or neuromuscular disorders.

Surgical Approaches

The diaphragm can be approached from the thorax or the abdomen. Either approach may be done with open or minimally invasive techniques.

Open Transthoracic Plication

Open transthoracic plication is the traditional approach to treat patients who are symptomatic and have diaphragm eventration or paralysis. A posterolateral thoracotomy is performed through the 6th,[42,43] 7th,[13,44,45] or 8th[46]

intercostal space. A variety of plication techniques have been described, including hand-sewn U stitches,[42,43,46,47] mattress sutures,[13,44] running sutures with or without pledgets, and stapling[48] techniques with or without mesh.[43,49] Another technique includes resecting the redundant portion of diaphragm and repairing the tissue in overlapping layers.[7,15] Open transthoracic plication has also been described as an approach to treating bilateral diaphragm paralysis.[50]

Multiple single-institution studies have demonstrated significant improvement in symptoms and respiratory function after open transthoracic plication.[42–46,51,52] In a study of 17 subjects who had unilateral paralysis, Graham and colleagues demonstrated that open transthoracic plication led to significant subjective improvement in dyspnea and orthopnea and PFT: FVC increased by 19% in the upright position and by 42% in the supine position.[45] Five to 10-year follow-up data was available for six subjects: durable improvements in dyspnea scores and PFT were observed.[13] In a study of 19 subjects, Higgs and colleagues also demonstrated durable improvements in dyspnea scores and PFT after open transthoracic plication at 5- to 10-year follow-up. Open transthoracic plication has demonstrated that plicating the diaphragm for symptomatic eventration or paralysis provides clear short- and long-term benefits. Unfortunately, open transthoracic plication is invasive, which can preclude the option of plication in patients who have multiple comorbidities. Consequently, alternative approaches to diaphragmatic plication have been developed to minimize the disadvantages of the open transthoracic approach.

Thoracoscopic Plication

Thoracoscopic plication can be performed using two ports with a mini-thoracotomy,[53,54] three ports,[12,55] or four ports.[56] Plication techniques including continuous sutures,[54,56] interrupted stitches,[12,55] or stapling[57] have been described. Single-institution studies have demonstrated improvement in dyspnea and PFT with thoracoscopic plication.[12,54,55] The largest series of thoracoscopic plication was published by Freeman and colleagues. In this report of 25 subjects who had unilateral diaphragm paralysis, thoracoscopic plication was successfully performed in 22 subjects, and 3 required conversion to thoracotomy. Follow-up at 6 months demonstrated a significant improvement in dyspnea scores and a significant increase in FVC (17%), FEV_1 (21%), functional residual capacity (FRC) (20%), and total lung capacity (TLC) (16%).

Thoracoscopic diaphragm plication is an excellent minimally invasive alternative to open transthoracic plication; mid-term follow-up data suggest that it is as effective as the open approach. Workspace limitation by the ribcage and the elevated hemidiaphragm is the main disadvantage of this approach.

Open Transabdominal Plication

Open transabdominal plication has been described for unilateral or bilateral diaphragmatic eventration or paralysis.[58] Little outcome data are available on the results of open transabdominal plication in adults. Advantages of an open transabdominal approach are access to both sides of the diaphragm and that it does not require selective ventilation. Additionally, a laparotomy is generally a less morbid incision than a thoracotomy. Disadvantages include an open approach and difficult access to the most posterior portion of the diaphragm.

Laparoscopic Plication

Laparoscopic diaphragm plication has been described in a single report of three patients by Hüttl and colleagues.[59] All patients improved clinically and by PFT parameters. Laparoscopic diaphragm plication is the preferred approach for diaphragm eventration or paralysis at the University of Minnesota.

Anesthesia
The procedure is performed under general anesthesia with a single-lumen endotracheal tube; selective ventilation is not necessary.

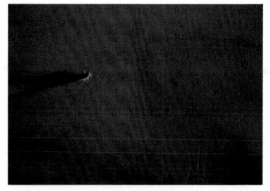

Fig. 2. The right hemidiaphragm is taut and displaced cranially from the pneumoperitoneum; a small perforation is made with electrocautery to induce a pneumothorax.

Position
Patients are in the supine position with abducted arms. The abdomen and lower lateral chest wall are prepared and draped to allow access for chest tube placement, a foot board is essential for steep Trendelenburg positioning.

Operative technique

(1) Ports: The authors place four 12-mm ports; two ports are placed along the midline for the camera and the assistant, and two working ports are placed in the ipsilateral upper quadrant (**Fig. 1**). The authors insufflate the abdomen with CO_2 at a pressure of 12 to 15 mmHg.

(2) Exposure: Steep reverse Trendelenburg positioning helps to optimize exposure of the posterior portion of the hemidiaphragm; for a right-sided plication, transection of the falciform ligament is useful for appropriate

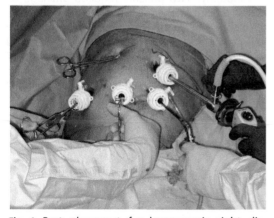

Fig. 1. Port placement for laparoscopic right diaphragm plication. The two operating ports are placed in the right upper quadrant approximately 2 cm above the level of the umbilicus. The two assistant ports are placed along the midline above the umbilicus; the costal margins have been marked with ink.

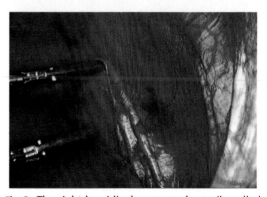

Fig. 3. The right hemidiaphragm can be easily pulled toward the abdominal cavity after inducing a pneumothorax. The diaphragm perforation is visible in the top left corner of the image.

access to the diaphragm. The thinned-out hemidiaphragm is taut and displaced cranially as a result of the pneumoperitoneum. The authors make a small perforation at the dome of the diaphragm with electrocautery (**Fig. 2**). The resultant pneumothorax allows the surgeon to easily pull the hemidiaphragm into the abdominal cavity for suturing (**Fig. 3**). To date, all patients have tolerated an ipsilateral pneumothorax well.

(3) Stitching: The authors use pledgeted U stitches (#2 nonabsorbable, braided suture, 31 mm curved needle) (**Fig. 4**). The posterior portion is plicated first in an anteroposterior direction followed by a plication line in lateromedial direction. This results in a T-shaped plication (**Fig. 5**). The initial perforation at the dome is closed with the plication.

(4) Tube thoracostomy: the authors place an 18- to 20-Fr chest tube in the ipsilateral chest at the end of the procedure.

Postoperative management

Patients should engage in intense pulmonary toilet to re-expand the lower lobe of the ipsilateral lung.

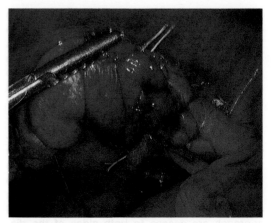

Fig. 5. The completed T-shaped plication.

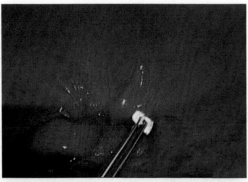

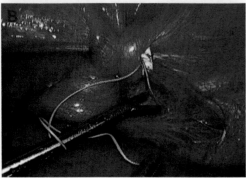

Fig. 4. (*A*) A row of pledgeted U stitches is first placed in posteroanterior direction. It is important to place stitches as far posteriorly as possible to achieve an effective plication. (*B*) Intracorporeal tying of a stitch. Notice the plication line emerging in the posteroanterior direction from behind the liver.

The chest tube remains in place until output is less than 200 mL/day; on occasion patients need to be discharged with the chest tube in place. Premature removal of the chest tube can lead to symptomatic pleural effusion. The immediate postoperative chest X ray should show that the plicated side is lower than the opposite side, one may see elevation of the contralateral hemidiaphragm; at 1 month both hemidiaphragms are at approximately the same level (**Fig. 6**). The authors monitor patients with the St. George's Respiratory Questionnaire (SGRQ),[60] PA/LAT chest X ray, and PFT at 1 month after discharge, and yearly thereafter.

Results

To date, the authors have performed laparoscopic plication on 18 patients with one conversion to thoracotomy. Two patients required drainage of a delayed ipsilateral pleural effusion. One- and 12-month follow-up revealed a significant improvement in SGRQ scores: 50% reduction in total score at 1 month that persisted at 12 months. PFT also improved significantly the FIFmax improved by a mean of 25% at 1 month and 45% at 12 months; FEV_1 improved by a mean of 12% and 18% respectively. These changes are comparable to the published results of open transthoracic plication and thoracoscopic plication.

Complications of Plication

Reported complications include pneumonia,[42,54] pleural effusions, abdominal compartment syndrome,[61] conversion to open (for minimally invasive approaches),[16] abdominal visceral injury, deep venous thrombosis,[12] pulmonary emboli,[46] and acute myocardial infarction.[46]

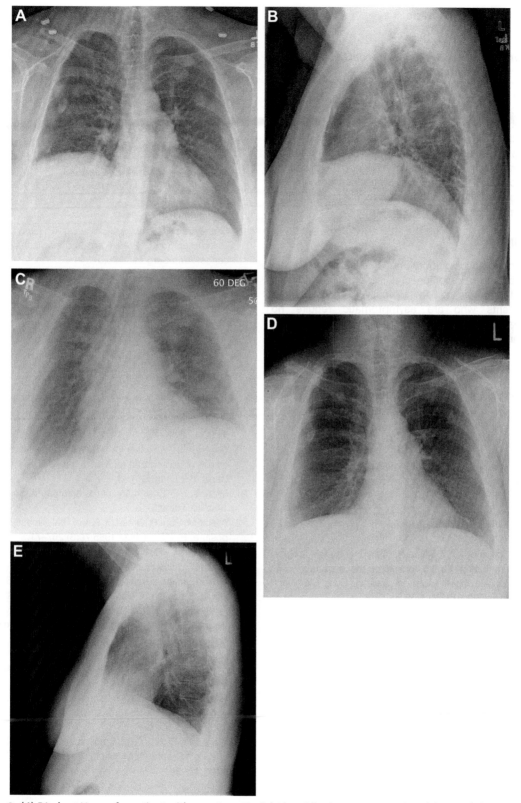

Fig. 6. (*A*) PA chest X ray of a patient with symptomatic right hemidiaphragm eventration. (*B*) Lateral chest X ray of a patient with symptomatic right hemidiaphragm eventration. (*C*) Immediate postoperative anteroposterior (AP) chest X ray of a patient after laparoscopic right hemidiaphragm plication; the right hemidiaphragm is lower than the left. (*D*) PA chest X ray 1 month after laparoscopic right hemidiaphragm plication; both sides of the diaphragm are at a similar level. (*E*) Lateral chest X ray 1 month after laparoscopic right hemidiaphragm plication; both sides of the diaphragm are at a similar level.

Comparison of Surgical Approaches for Diaphragm Plication

No direct comparison of the various diaphragm plication techniques has been performed. Published results suggest that results of transthoracic and transabdominal approaches are comparable. Currently, plication should be attempted by minimally invasive techniques, since the morbidity is probably less than with an open approach. The choice of thoracoscopic or laparoscopic plication is mostly the surgeon's preference.

SUMMARY

Symptomatic diaphragmatic eventration is an uncommon condition and is sometimes impossible to distinguish clinically from paralysis. Patients who are asymptomatic require no treatment; patients who are symptomatic benefit significantly from diaphragm plication. The choice of plication approach is dependent upon the expertise of the surgeon.

REFERENCES

1. Deslauriers J. Eventration of the diaphragm. Chest Surg Clin N Am 1998;8(2):315–30.
2. Chin EF, Lynn RB. Surgery of eventration of the diaphragm. J Thorac Surg 1956;32(1):6–14.
3. Christensen P. Eventration of the diaphragm. Thorax 1959;14:311–9.
4. McNamara JJ, Paulson DL, Urschel HC Jr, et al. Eventration of the diaphragm. Surgery 1968;64(6): 1013–21.
5. Schumpelick V, Steinau G, Schlüper I, et al. Surgical embryology and anatomy of the diaphragm with surgical applications [xi review]. Surg Clin North Am 2000;80(1):213–39.
6. Thomas TV. Nonparalytic eventration of the diaphragm. J Thorac Cardiovasc Surg 1968;55(4): 586–93.
7. Thomas TV. Congenital eventration of the diaphragm. Ann Thorac Surg 1970;10(2):180–92.
8. Riley EA. Idiopathic diaphragmatic paralysis; a report of eight cases. Am J Med 1962;32:404–16.
9. Efthimiou J, Butler J, Woodham C, et al. Diaphragm paralysis following cardiac surgery: role of phrenic nerve cold injury. Ann Thorac Surg 1991;52(4): 1005–8.
10. Curtis JJ, Nawarawong W, Walls JT, et al. Elevated hemidiaphragm after cardiac operations: incidence, prognosis, and relationship to the use of topical ice slush. Ann Thorac Surg 1989;48(6):764–8.
11. Markand ON, Moorthy SS, Mahomed Y, et al. Postoperative phrenic nerve palsy in patients with open-heart surgery. Ann Thorac Surg 1985;39(1): 68–73.
12. Freeman RK, Wozniak TC, Fitzgerald EB. Functional and physiologic results of video-assisted thoracoscopic diaphragm plication in adult patients with unilateral diaphragm paralysis. Ann Thorac Surg 2006;81(5):1853–7 [discussion: 1857].
13. Graham DR, Kaplan D, Evans CC, et al. Diaphragmatic plication for unilateral diaphragmatic paralysis: a 10-year experience. Ann Thorac Surg 1990; 49(2):248–51 [discussion: 252].
14. Obara H, Hoshina H, Iwai S, et al. Eventration of the diaphragm in infants and children. Acta Paediatr Scand 1987;76(4):654–8.
15. Shah-Mirany J, Schmitz GL, Watson RR. Eventration of the diaphragm. Physiologic and surgical significance. Arch Surg 1968;96(5):844–50.
16. Gibson GJ. Diaphragmatic paresis: pathophysiology, clinical features, and investigation. Thorax 1989;44(11):960–70.
17. Ridyard JB, Stewart RM. Regional lung function in unilateral diaphragmatic paralysis. Thorax 1976; 31(4):438–42.
18. McCredie M, Lovejoy FW, Kaltreider NL. Pulmonary function in diaphragmatic paralysis. Thorax 1962; 17:213–7.
19. Hoover CF. The functions of the diaphragm and their diagnostic significance. Arch Intern Med 1913;12: 214–24.
20. Grinman S, Whitelaw WA. Pattern of breathing in a case of generalized respiratory muscle weakness. Chest 1983;84(6):770–2.
21. Michelson E. Eventration of the diaphragm. Surgery 1961;49:410–22.
22. Allen SM, Hunt B, Green M. Fall in vital capacity with posture. Br J Dis Chest 1985;79(3):267–71.
23. Clague HW, Hall DR. Effect of posture on lung volume: airway closure and gas exchange in hemidiaphragmatic paralysis. Thorax 1979;34(4):523–6.
24. Gould L, Kaplan S, McElhinney AJ, et al. A method for the production of hemidiaphragmatic paralysis. Its application to the study of lung function in normal man. Am Rev Respir Dis 1967;96(4):812–4.
25. Wynn-Williams N. Hemidiaphragmatic paralysis and paresis of unknown aetiology without any marked rise in level. Thorax 1954;9:299–303.
26. Gierada DS, Slone RM, Fleishman MJ. Imaging evaluation of the diaphragm. Chest Surg Clin N Am 1998;8(2):237–80.
27. Alexander C. Diaphragm movements and the diagnosis of diaphragmatic paralysis. Clin Radiol 1966; 17(1):79–83.
28. Houston JG, Fleet M, Cowan MD, et al. Comparison of ultrasound with fluoroscopy in the assessment of suspected hemidiaphragmatic movement abnormality. Clin Radiol 1995;50(2):95–8.
29. Gottesman E, McCool FD. Ultrasound evaluation of the paralyzed diaphragm. Am J Respir Crit Care Med 1997;155(5):1570–4.

30. Summerhill EM, El-Sameed YA, Glidden TJ, et al. Monitoring recovery from diaphragm paralysis with ultrasound. Chest 2008;133(3):737–43.

31. Slone RM, Gierada DS. Radiology of pulmonary emphysema and lung volume reduction surgery. Semin Thorac Cardiovasc Surg 1996;8(1):61–82.

32. Wilcox PG, Pardy RL. Diaphragmatic weakness and paralysis. Lung 1989;167(6):323–41.

33. Miller JM, Moxham J, Green M. The maximal sniff in the assessment of diaphragm function in man. Clin Sci (Lond) 1985;69(1):91–6.

34. Laporta D, Grassino A. Assessment of transdiaphragmatic pressure in humans. J Appl Physiol 1985; 58(5):1469–76.

35. Markand ON, Kincaid JC, Pourmand RA, et al. Electrophysiologic evaluation of diaphragm by transcutaneous phrenic nerve stimulation. Neurology 1984; 34(5):604–14.

36. Bellemare F, Bigland-Ritchie B. Assessment of human diaphragm strength and activation using phrenic nerve stimulation. Respir Physiol 1984; 58(3):263–77.

37. Morrison JMW. Eventration of the diaphragm due to unilateral phrenic nerve paralysis. Arch Radiol Electrotherap 1923;28:72–5.

38. Chervin RD, Guilleminault C. Diaphragm pacing for respiratory insufficiency. J Clin Neurophysiol 1997; 14(5):369–77.

39. Glenn WW, Holcomb WG, Hogan J, et al. Diaphragm pacing by radiofrequency transmission in the treatment of chronic ventilatory insufficiency. Present status. J Thorac Cardiovasc Surg 1973;66(4): 505–20.

40. DiMarco AF. Restoration of respiratory muscle function following spinal cord injury. Review of electrical and magnetic stimulation techniques. Respir Physiol Neurobiol 2005;147(2–3):273–87.

41. Gayan-Ramirez G, Gosselin N, Troosters T, et al. Functional recovery of diaphragm paralysis: a long-term follow-up study. Respir Med 2008; 102(5):690–8.

42. Kuniyoshi Y, Yamashiro S, Miyagi K, et al. Diaphragmatic plication in adult patients with diaphragm paralysis after cardiac surgery. Ann Thorac Cardiovasc Surg 2004;10(3):160–6.

43. Simansky DA, Paley M, Refaely Y, et al. Diaphragm plication following phrenic nerve injury: a comparison of paediatric and adult patients. Thorax 2002; 57(7):613–6.

44. Wright CD, Williams JG, Ogilvie CM, et al. Results of diaphragmatic plication for unilateral diaphragmatic paralysis. J Thorac Cardiovasc Surg 1985;90(2): 195–8.

45. Higgs SM, Hussain A, Jackson M, et al. Long term results of diaphragmatic plication for unilateral diaphragm paralysis. Eur J Cardiothorac Surg 2002; 21(2):294–7.

46. Versteegh MI, Braun J, Voigt PG, et al. Diaphragm plication in adult patients with diaphragm paralysis leads to long-term improvement of pulmonary function and level of dyspnea. Eur J Cardiothorac Surg 2007;32(3):449–56.

47. Schwartz MZ, Filler RM. Plication of the diaphragm for symptomatic phrenic nerve paralysis. J Pediatr Surg 1978;13(3):259–63.

48. Maxson T, Robertson R, Wagner CW. An improved method of diaphragmatic plication. Surg Gynecol Obstet 1993;177(6):620–1.

49. Di Giorgio A, Cardini CL, Sammartino P, et al. Dual-layer sandwich mesh repair in the treatment of major diaphragmatic eventration in an adult. J Thorac Cardiovasc Surg 2006;132(1):187–9.

50. Stolk J, Versteegh MI. Long-term effect of bilateral plication of the diaphragm. Chest 2000;117(3):786–9.

51. Ciccolella DE, Daly BD, Celli BR. Improved diaphragmatic function after surgical plication for unilateral diaphragmatic paralysis. Am Rev Respir Dis 1992;146(3):797–9.

52. Ribet M, Linder JL. Plication of the diaphragm for unilateral eventration or paralysis. Eur J Cardiothorac Surg 1992;6(7):357–60.

53. Mouroux J, Padovani B, Poirier NC, et al. Technique for the repair of diaphragmatic eventration. Ann Thorac Surg 1996;62(3):905–7.

54. Mouroux J, Venissac N, Leo F, et al. Surgical treatment of diaphragmatic eventration using video-assisted thoracic surgery: a prospective study. Ann Thorac Surg 2005;79(1):308–12.

55. Suzumura Y, Terada Y, Sonobe M, et al. A case of unilateral diaphragmatic eventration treated by plication with thoracoscopic surgery. Chest 1997; 112(2):530–2.

56. Hwang Z, Shin JS, Cho YH, et al. A simple technique for the thoracoscopic plication of the diaphragm. Chest 2003;124(1):376–8.

57. Moon SW, Wang YP, Kim YW, et al. Thoracoscopic plication of diaphragmatic eventration using endostaplers. Ann Thorac Surg 2000;70(1):299–300.

58. Kizilcan F, Tanyel FC, Hiçsönmez A, et al. The long-term results of diaphragmatic plication. J Pediatr Surg 1993;28(1):42–4.

59. Hüttl TP, Wichmann MW, Reichart B, et al. Laparoscopic diaphragmatic plication: long-term results of a novel surgical technique for postoperative phrenic nerve palsy. Surg Endosc 2004;18(3): 547–51.

60. Jones PW, Quirk FH, Baveystock CM, et al. A self-complete measure of health status for chronic airflow limitation. The St. George's Respiratory Questionnaire. Am Rev Respir Dis 1992;145(6):1321–7.

61. Phadnis J, Pilling JE, Evans TW, et al. Abdominal compartment syndrome: a rare complication of plication of the diaphragm. Ann Thorac Surg 2006; 82(1):334–6.

Tumors of the Diaphragm

Min Peter Kim, MD, Wayne L. Hofstetter, MD*

KEYWORDS

• Diaphragm tumor • Cyst • Lipoma • Sarcoma

A tumor of the diaphragm, a very rare event, was first described in 1868 by Grancher, who found a fibroma of the diaphragm during autopsy. To date, only 144 cases of primary tumors of the diaphragm have been reported in the literature.[1–24] Drewes and Willmann[25] reported the first series of 49 cases of diaphragm tumors in 1955. In 1965, Wiener and Chou[26] added 22 more cases to the literature, thus increasing the collective count to 71 diaphragmatic tumors. More recently, multiple investigators have contributed small descriptive series and case reports, none larger than the original series described by Drewes, underscoring the rarity of these tumors and the lack of knowledge about them.[27–29]

Primary tumors of the diaphragm are classified as benign or malignant. The most common benign lesions of the diaphragm are diaphragmatic cysts, with 38 cases in the literature, and lipomas, with 13 cases in the literature. The most common malignant primary lesions of the diaphragm are rhabdomyosarcoma, with 15 cases reported in the literature, and fibrosarcoma, with 9 cases reported. Analysis of the 144 cases of diaphragm tumors reported in the literature shows that the tumors affect slightly more females (54%) than males (46%). The average age of presentation was 40 years old with range of 28 days from birth to 80 years of age. Fifty-eight percent of the tumors reported in the literature were benign tumors of the diaphragm. Tumors were equally distributed between the left and right side of the diaphragm. The most common presenting symptoms were chest pain or abdominal pain. Only 15% of patients with benign tumors and 11% of patients with malignant tumors presented incidentally. Some of the reported tumors were found during autopsy.

In addition to the primary tumors of the diaphragm, there are metastatic lesions to the diaphragm, which can be classified as benign, such as endometriosis, or malignant lesions. Malignant tumors can also involve the diaphragm via direct extension from another source. Metastatic tumors and tumors involving the diaphragm by direct extension make up the vast majority of tumors typically encountered by a thoracic surgeon.

BENIGN PRIMARY TUMOR
Diaphragm Cysts

The most common benign lesion of the diaphragm is a cyst, most often either a mesothelial cyst or a bronchogenic cyst. Mesothelial cysts are congenital lesions arising from coelomic remnants, which can be found in the adrenal gland, ovary, falciform ligament, spleen, vaginal process of the testicle, mesentery, and, rarely, the diaphragm.[30] The cyst is seen in children and adults. Two case series described children (3.5–14 years) who presented with nonspecific abdominal complaints,[19,30] while another described patients who presented without any symptoms.[31] Ultrasound was the initial diagnostic study for children and this showed a thin-walled cystic structure.[19,30] The CT scan showed homogeneous, nonenhancing, well-defined cysts of water density,[19,30] while MRI showed a thin-walled cystic structure attached to the diaphragm.[19,30] The diagnosis of mesothelial cyst of the diaphragm was typically based on the imaging. Some patients underwent percutaneous aspiration of the cyst, which yielded clear yellowish fluid consistent with mesothelial cyst.[30] Among children with mesothelial cyst, some patients had surgical resection,

Division of Thoracic and Cardiovascular Surgery, MD Anderson Cancer Center, The University of Texas, 1515 Holcombe Boulevard, Unit 445, Houston, TX 77030-4009, USA
* Corresponding author.
E-mail address: whofstetter@mdanderson.org (W.L. Hofstetter).

Thorac Surg Clin 19 (2009) 521–529
doi:10.1016/j.thorsurg.2009.08.007

which confirmed the diagnosis. However, a report by Akinci and colleagues[19,30] on 11 patients followed with serial ultrasound showed regression or complete resolution in 6 patients and no change in size for 5 patients (follow-up 5 months to 6 years) indicating that an aggressive surgical approach is not always necessary. Moreover, this study reported on cysts successfully treated with ethanol sclerotherapy. Five patients underwent injection of cyst volume with 95% ethanol, which lead to resolution of the cyst in all patients.[30] Presentation of cyst in adults was even more uncommon than in children and was most often symptomatic, with patients complaining of chest pain, upper abdominal discomfort, and dyspnea.[26,31–33] All of these patients underwent surgical resection of the cysts. Extrapolation of the literature would suggest that asymptomatic cysts could be managed conservatively and symptomatic cysts approached surgically or percutaneously.

Bronchogenic cysts are foregut-derived developmental anomalies usually located in the mediastinum or lung parenchyma. These are aberrant buds from the tracheobronchial tree that rest in an abnormal location.[34] There are isolated case reports of bronchogenic cysts of the diaphragm.[12,26,35] The cyst wall is lined with ciliated pseudostratified columnar epithelium, the sine qua non of bronchogenic cyst. The histology is similar to that of the bronchial wall and the uncomplicated cyst is filled with viscous mucoid material.[35] Some patients had no symptoms,[12,34] but most presented with cough, discomfort, pain, or hiccups.[26,35] Symptomatic patients had very large cysts causing compression of surrounding structures. The lesion may be detected on chest radiograph as a bulging mass over the diaphragm,[34] while CT would reveal linear and nodular calcifications along the cyst wall with soft tissue density within the lesion.[34,36] Ultrasound shows a hypoechoic lesion[34,36] and an MRI shows a fluid-containing lesion.[36] It is difficult to confirm the exact diagnosis from preoperative imaging.[12,35,36] Some benign cysts of the diaphragm can be mistaken for cystic tumors of the liver on CT imaging.

Little is known about the natural history of bronchogenic cysts of the diaphragm as most of those that have been described were resected by laparotomy,[36] video-assisted thoracoscopy,[12] or laparoscopy.[35] In most cases, the cystic lesions were removed to establish a diagnosis, to alleviate symptoms, or to rule out intracystic carcinoma.[34] However, there are no reports of intracystic carcinoma of the diaphragm in the literature. Enucleation or complete resection have both been described, and the ability to primarily repair or patch repair the remaining defect in the diaphragm

after resection is based on the size of the tumor. Overall, benign cysts can be observed. However, the cyst should be removed if it is symptomatic or there is a question of the diagnosis.

Another reason to consider resection of a cystic diaphragm lesion is when there is concern that the lesion may be a hydatid cyst. A hydatid cyst results from the tapeworm *Echinococcus granulosus*, which is prevalent in Mediterranean countries.[10] The eggs of the tapeworm excreted by carnivores may infect various species of intermediate hosts, such as sheep, cattle, deer, and humans.[3] The tapeworm is usually found in the liver because the embryo hexacanth enters through the intestine into the portal system and forms cysts in the liver.[10] The tapeworm then can travel to the lung and the spleen, which are the other two common sites of the disease. It is rarely found in the diaphragm (incidence is about 1%). It travels to the diaphragm through the vascular system or direct extension from the liver or the lung.[10] Most patients present with pain[9,18]; there is even a reported case of ruptured diaphragmatic hydatid cyst.[3] The diagnosis can be made by indirect hemagglutination test, which is usually positive for hydatid cyst. Ultrasound shows a cyst with multiple vesicles. A CT scan would show a mass lesion with solid and cystic components.[3] MRI shows a cystic structure with multiple vesicles inside.[18] The treatment is careful, complete surgical resection, usually cystotomy and removal of daughter cyst and the germinative membrane, then excision of most of the pericyst, followed by diaphragmatic repair. After resection of hydatid cysts, patients should be given albendazole for a period of time.[18] All three reports of confirmed hydatid cyst of the diaphragm are from Greece and Turkey.[3,7,18] However, for patients with a cystic lesion of the diaphragm who have a travel history to endemic areas, this disease should be included in the differential diagnosis.

Lipomatous Tumors of the Diaphragm

Lipomas of the diaphragm are the most common benign solid tumors of the diaphragm. Lipomas are soft encapsulated fatty tumors. There are two forms of diaphragmatic lipomas: sessile lipomas, which develop from subpleural mature fatty tissue, and hourglass-shaped lipomas, which develop from embryologically undifferentiated tissue.[37,38] Most patients with lipoma are asymptomatic. However, patients with a large lipoma might present with cough, pain, or dyspnea. The best diagnostic test is a CT scan, which shows a lesion with Hounsfield units consistent with adipose tissue (**Fig. 1**).[37,39] Sometimes, a primary lipoma of the diaphragm is mistaken for Bochdalek hernia. A potentially distinguishing CT finding is that the integrity of the diaphragm is complete with lipoma while Bochdalek hernias present with a V-shaped discontinuity of the diaphragm.[20,39]

There is one case report of liposarcoma in the literature. The CT appearance of the liposarcoma of the diaphragm was a heterogeneous enhancing solid lesion with fat and septae of connective tissue. The lesion was removed, confirming the histology as liposarcoma.[40] Some suggest that patients with small incidentally recognized lipomas can be observed.[37] However, in symptomatic patients or asymptomatic patients with concern for liposarcoma, the lesion should be resected.[39,40] There may be no defining features of one over the other and differentiating lipoma from liposarcoma may require histologic examination of the lesion.

Other Benign Primary Tumors

Some other benign tumors of the diaphragm reported in the literature are listed in **Table 1**. In case reports and descriptive series, most patients presented with symptoms of pain or dyspnea. Other cases were found incidentally during an autopsy. In patients who presented with symptoms, a CT scan was obtained that showed a lesion in the diaphragm, although it was often hard to distinguish from an intra-abdominal or pleural lesion. In most cases, the lesion was resected and the final pathology confirmed a benign tumor of the diaphragm.

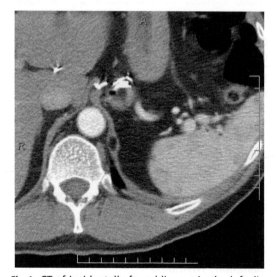

Fig. 1. CT of incidentally found lipoma in the left diaphragmatic crus. (*Courtesy of* B. Sabloff, MD, Houston, TX.)

BENIGN METASTATIC LESIONS TO THE DIAPHRAGM
Endometriosis

Endometriosis is an ectopic growth of endometrial stromal and glandular tissue outside the uterine cavity.[41] It is typically found on the ovaries, uterine ligaments, bladder, and bowel. It is rarely found on the diaphragm.[41] The theory behind the implantation of endometrial contents in the pelvis and the abdomen is retrograde menstruation. Most patients present with upper abdominal pain or shoulder pain while some patients are asymptomatic.[42] Patients can also present with catamenial pneumothorax. About 80% of patients with thoracic endometriosis defined by presence of endometrial tissues on the lung, pleura, or the diaphragm present with catamenial pneumothorax, where patient's pneumothorax occurs within 72 hours after menstruation.[43] Patients may also have symptoms of chest pain or shortness of breath. Rarely, hemothorax or hemoptysis is present. Initial diagnosis can be confused with pulmonary embolism until imaging suggests otherwise.[43] Diagnostic imaging via a CT scan may identify a mass, but it often cannot determine its nature. However, MRI may be able to diagnose endometriosis by appearance of hemorrhage within endometriomata and by one or more surrounding low-intensity rings.[44] For unknown reasons, diaphragm involvement is typically on the right.[43] Ultimately, the best diagnostic test is either video-assisted thoracoscopy or laparoscopy.[43] The first-line treatment for endometriosis is medical therapy with hormone suppression. Ablation or resection is reserved for symptomatic patients or asymptomatic patients who are worried about progression of disease and who have failed medical therapy.[42] The best surgical option is resection with primary closure,[41,43] but small lesions may be vaporized using hydrodissection and carbon dioxide laser or cavitational ultrasonographic surgical aspirator.[42]

MALIGNANT PRIMARY TUMORS OF THE DIAPHRAGM
Rhabdomyosarcoma

Rhabdomyosarcoma is a malignant tumor arising from embryonal mesenchymal cells with potential to differentiate into skeletal muscle cells. There are four histologic classes of rhabdomyosarcoma: pleomorphic, alveolar, botryoid, and embryonal.[4] Embryonal is the most common type (58%).[45] It can occur at any site, but is usually found in the head and neck region (42%), urogenital tract

Table 1
Benign primary tumors of the diaphragm

Tumor Type	Number of Reported Cases	Reference
Cyst	38	Wiener,[26] Chang,[12] Zugel,[35] Elemen,[2] Anile,[14] Rozenblit,[36] Dervisoglu,[3] Eren,[18] Akinci,[30] Marinis[7]
Lipoma	13	Wiener,[26] Papachristos,[39] Cheon,[11] Oyar,[20,37] Sen[5]
Neurofibroma	5	Wiener,[26] Cada[13]
Angiofibroma	3	Wiener[26]
Fibroma	3	Wiener[26]
Hemangioma	3	Ohsaki,[65] Kaniklides,[23] Kono[8]
Schwannoma	3	Wiener,[26] Ohba[1]
Chondroma	2	Wiener,[26] Itakura[66]
Hemangioendothelioma	2	Wiener,[26] Weksler[27]
Angioleiomyoma	1	Van Rijn[22]
Endothelioma	1	Wiener[26]
Fibrolymphangioma	1	Wiener[26]
Fibroangioendothelioma	1	Wiener[26]
Fibromyoma	1	Wiener[26]
Hamartoma	1	Wiener[26]
Leiomyoma	1	Wiener[26]
Lymphangioma	1	Wiener[26]
Myofibroma	1	Cada[13]
Rhabdomyofibroma	1	Wiener[26]

(34%), or extremities (11%). It is very rarely found in the diaphragm. Much of what is known about rhabdomyosarcoma is derived from data related to disease found other than at the diaphragm. Of the handful described within the diaphragm, most patients were asymptomatic but some presented with chest pain, cough, dyspnea, dysphagia, or abdominal mass.[24] On diagnostic CT scan, a rhabdomyosarcoma of the diaphragm appears as a heterogeneous, enhancing diaphragmatic mass. Histologic diagnosis is generally made by image-guided biopsy. Recommendation for treatment is typically resection with adjuvant chemoradiation. For larger tumors, induction chemotherapy followed by surgical resection and adjuvant radiation has been described.[46,47]

Leiomyosarcoma

Leiomyosarcoma is most frequently found in the uterus and gastrointestinal tract.[48,49] It is rarely found in the diaphragm. Most of the patients with diaphragm involvement described in the literature were asymptomatic but abdominal pain was the most common symptomatic presentation. On CT scan, a leiomyosarcoma appears as

a heterogeneous mass with low density and MRI shows a mass with low signal intensity at T1 and isointensity at T2. Surgical resection is considered the best treatment. There are no known therapeutic benefits from chemotherapy or radiotherapy in resectable lesions.[48]

Other Malignant Primary Tumors of the Diaphragm

Table 2 lists other primary malignant lesions that have been found on the diaphragm. Most of the other malignant primary tumors of the diaphragm should be treated based on tumor type found on biopsy and resectability on imaging. When formulating a treatment plan for these extremely rare lesions, one should use the knowledge of a tumor's historical response to chemotherapy, radiotherapy, and surgery extrapolated from similar histology at other primary sites.[13]

MALIGNANT METASTATIC TUMORS TO THE DIAPHRAGM
Malignant Thymoma

Thymomas are rare malignant epithelial tumors occurring within the anterior mediastinum.[50] The

Table 2
Malignant primary tumors of the diaphragm

Tumor Type	Number of Reported Cases	Reference
Rhabdomyosarcoma	15	Mandal,[28] Cada,[13] Vade,[47] Chatterjee,[67] Wiener,[26] Weksler,[27] Deniz[4]
Fibrosarcoma	9	Wiener,[26] Weksler[27]
Neurofibrosarcoma	3	Wiener,[26] Weksler[27]
Sarcoma, undifferentiated	3	Wiener[26]
Yolk sac tumor	3	Cada,[13] Weksler[27]
Extraskeletal Ewing's sarcoma	2	Eroglu,[17] Song[68]
Fibromyosarcoma	2	Wiener[26]
Angiosarcoma	1	Moriya[6]
Chondrosarcoma	1	Weksler[27]
Desmoid tumor	1	Soysai[69]
Germ cell tumor	1	Traubici[15]
Hemangiopericytoma	1	Weksler[27]
Liposarcoma	1	Froehner[40]
Pheochromocytoma	1	Jacob[21]
Malignant fibrous histiocytoma	1	Tanaka[70]
Malignant hemangiopericytoma	1	Wiener[26]
Malignant schwannoma	1	Kumbasar[16]
Mesothelioma	1	Wiener[26]
Mixed cell sarcoma	1	Wiener[26]
Myoblastic sarcoma	1	Wiener[26]
Myosarcoma	1	Wiener[26]
Vascular sarcoma	1	Wiener[26]

histologic patterns seen are spindle cell and medullary thymoma, mixed pattern of lymphocyte and lymphocyte-rich thymoma, and thymoma resembling the normal thymic epithelial cells with subtypes characterized by increasing epithelial/lymphocyte ratio. Thymic tumors can form "drop metastases," tumors that form within the pleural space and that are thought to be secondary to direct shedding of tumor cells. Drop metastases on the diaphragm, although strictly speaking represent advanced disease, are often resectable and removal may provide the patient with the best opportunity for a cure. Mineo and Biancari[51] described a series of seven patients who had recurrent thymoma. For three of these patients, the thymoma was located in the diaphragm. Each of these three patients had aggressive surgical resection, which provided a prolonged disease-free survival. Other reports describe benefit from resection of thymoma and the drop metastasis after induction chemotherapy.[52–54] Diagnosis is most reliably made by transthoracic needle biopsy or thoracoscopy.

Ovarian Cancer

Advanced ovarian cancer can often involve the peritoneal surface of the diaphragm. Standard initial therapy for patients with advanced ovarian cancer is primary surgical cytoreduction. In cases that involve the diaphragm, diaphragm stripping may achieve optimal cytoreduction. However, when the ovarian cancer penetrates the muscle with a large amount of disease, a full diaphragmatic resection with primary repair has been advocated.[55] There are some case reports of patients who benefitted from an en bloc resection of the diaphragm and the lung if they were involved.[56]

DIRECT EXTENSION OF MALIGNANCY TO THE DIAPHRAGM

Many types of intra-abdominal malignancy with direct involvement of the diaphragm may result in the thoracic surgeon's participation. Tumors arising from the abdominal contents or retroperitoneum, such as hepatic, renal, or retroperitoneal malignancies, can involve the diaphragm. Treatment of these lesions is generally not precluded by the direct extension into the diaphragm and en bloc resection of the mass along with the diaphragm is common. Typically, there is enough residual diaphragm to repair primarily. However, if there is concern about tension on the repair, it is advisable to consider using some type of patch for reconstruction. Of particular interest to the thoracic surgeon are malignancies commonly seen within the thorax that may directly invade into the diaphragm.

Lung Cancer Invading the Diaphragm

Invasion of the diaphragm from lung cancer is a very rare occurrence that takes place in only 0.5% of lung cancers. Lung cancer invading the diaphragm without lymph node involvement (T3N0M0) is probably best classified as stage IIb disease, as the 5-year survival in resected patients is reported as 33%.[57–59] Factors that reduce survival in this group of patients include the inability to achieve a complete resection, deep invasion of the diaphragm compared with patients with shallow invasion, and the presence of any lymph node involvement combined with diaphragm involvement.[58] Optimal treatment for resectable patients with involvement of the diaphragm would be en bloc resection of involved lung and the diaphragm with appropriate diaphragm reconstruction.[60]

Mesothelioma

Malignant mesothelioma, a rare tumor of the pleura, involves the diaphragm through direct extension. In early stages, patients typically present with dyspnea. Then, as disease progresses, patients may also complain of chest pain. The diagnosis is often made by thoracentesis as most patients have pleural fluid, which is positive for malignancy in 30% to 50% of patients. Diagnostic imaging with CT and positron emission tomography scans is helpful in characterizing the tumor and its stage. Tumor may involve the diaphragmatic parietal pleura or invade transmurally through the diaphragm. The treatment is based on the stage of the tumor. Any sign of invasion through the diaphragm into the abdomen seen on MRI or laparoscopy precludes resection. Tumors limited to the hemithorax can be resected by pleurectomy-decortication or extrapleural pneumonectomy. In extrapleural pneumonectomy, the entire diaphragm is removed and reconstructed with foreign material. In pleurectomy, the diaphragm is resected only if it is involved. No clear evidence demonstrates that one operation is better than the other. While some studies suggest that pleurectomy and decortication may provide improved survival with fewer complications, the evidence may be tainted by selection bias.[61,62]

Esophageal Cancer to the Diaphragm

Local extension of esophageal cancer into the diaphragm is correctly described as a T4 tumor. Although the survival for patients with T4 cancer is typically considered poor, primary extension of a transmural esophageal tumor into the diaphragm does not preclude resection and long-term survival can be achieved. At most centers, patients with locally advanced esophageal cancer receive combined chemoradiotherapy before surgery. The diaphragm resection would be included as part of a radical esophagectomy.

RECONSTRUCTION

Tumors excised from the diaphragm result in a defect that must be repaired. A surgeon experienced in thoracic surgery and resection of the diaphragm should participate in operations that involve resection and reconstruction of the diaphragm. Lack of appropriate repair can lead to life-threatening complications. A poorly reconstructed diaphragm can result in symptomatic atelectasis and/or recurrent pneumonia if the diaphragm is repaired with a patch that is too large. Alternatively, if too much tension is placed on a repair, it can ultimately break down and lead to diaphragmatic hernia with potential for serious complications. This can be of rapid or insidious onset and it is wise to suggest long-term radiographic follow-up for any patient who has had diaphragm resection. Options for reconstruction include various prosthetic materials suitable for diaphragm reconstruction.[63] Also, some literature supports the use of tissue flaps, particularly when there is concern for leaving behind a foreign material with risk of infection/erosion. Some of the flaps that have been described include transversus abduminus/internal oblique muscle, external oblique muscle, latissimus dorsi muscle, and omentum.[64]

SUMMARY

Primary tumors of the diaphragm are rare. The most common benign cystic lesions of the diaphragm are bronchogenic or mesothelial cysts, while the most common benign solid lesion is a lipoma. Benign tumors of the diaphragm are resected if they are symptomatic or if there is a doubt about the diagnosis. The most common primary malignant lesion is rhabdomyosarcoma. Malignant tumors are treated based on histology and often with chemotherapy and/or radiation along with surgical resection if feasible. Endometriosis, a benign process that metastasizes to the diaphragm, is typically treated medically; surgical ablation or resection is considered only after failed conservative treatment. Surgical resection of metastatic malignant tumors, such as ovarian cancer and thymoma, as well as malignancies affecting the diaphragm by direct extension, such as mesothelioma, lung, and esophageal cancer, may provide some survival advantage.

REFERENCES

1. Ohba T, Shoji F, Kometani T, et al. Schwannoma in the peridiaphragm. Gen Thorac Cardiovasc Surg 2008;56(9):453–5.
2. Elemen L, Tugay M, Tugay S, et al. Bronchogenic cyst of the right hemidiaphragm mimicking a hydatid cyst of the liver: report of the first pediatric case. Pediatr Surg Int 2008;24(8):957–9.
3. Dervisoglu E, Topcu S, Liman ST, et al. Spontaneous rupture of a giant diaphragmatic hydatid cyst into the intrapleural space. Med Princ Pract 2008;17(1):86–8.
4. Deniz PP, Kalac N, Ucoluk GO, et al. A rare tumor of the diaphragm: pleomorphic rhabdomyosarcoma. Ann Thorac Surg 2008;85(5):1802–5.
5. Sen S, Discigil B, Badak I, et al. Lipoma of the diaphragm: a rare presentation. Ann Thorac Surg 2007;83(6):2203–5.
6. Moriya Y, Sugawara T, Arai M, et al. Bilateral massive bloody pleurisy complicated by angiosarcoma. Intern Med 2007;46(3):125–8.
7. Marinis A, Fragulidis G, Karapanos K, et al. Subcutaneous extension of a large diaphragmatic hydatid cyst. World J Gastroenterol 2006;12(44):7210–2.
8. Kono R, Terasaki H, Fujimoto K, et al. Venous hemangioma arising from the diaphragm: a case report of computed tomography and magnetic resonance imaging findings. J Thorac Imaging 2006;21(3):231–4.
9. Isik AF, Sagay S, Ciftci A. Diaphragmatic hydatid disease. Acta Chir Belg 2006;106(1):96–7.
10. Di Carlo I, Toro A, Sparatore F, et al. Isolated hydatid cyst of the diaphragm without liver or lung involvement: a case report. Acta Chir Belg 2006;106(5):599–601.
11. Cheon JS, You YK, Kim JG, et al. Diaphragmatic lipoma in a 4-year-old girl: a case report. J Pediatr Surg 2006;41(1):e37–9.
12. Chang YC, Chen JS, Chang YL, et al. Video-assisted thoracoscopic excision of intradiaphragmatic bronchogenic cysts: two cases. J Laparoendosc Adv Surg Tech A 2006;16(5):489–92.
13. Cada M, Gerstle JT, Traubici J, et al. Approach to diagnosis and treatment of pediatric primary tumors of the diaphragm. J Pediatr Surg 2006;41(10):1722–6.
14. Anile M, Di Stasio M, Vitolo D, et al. Intradiaphragmatic bronchogenic cyst. Eur J Cardiothorac Surg 2006;29(5):839.
15. Traubici J, Daneman A, Hayes-Jordan A, et al. Primary germ cell tumor of the diaphragm. J Pediatr Surg 2004;39(10):1578–80.
16. Kumbasar U, Enon S, Osman Tokat A, et al. An uncommon tumor of the diaphragm malignant schwannoma. Interact Cardiovasc Thorac Surg 2004;3(2):384–5.
17. Eroglu A, Kurkcuoglu IC, Karaoglanoglu N, et al. Extraskeletal Ewing sarcoma of the diaphragm presenting with hemothorax. Ann Thorac Surg 2004;78(2):715–7.
18. Eren S, Ulku R, Tanrikulu AC, et al. Primary giant hydatid cyst of the diaphragm. Ann Thorac Cardiovasc Surg 2004;10(2):118–9.
19. Esparza Estaun J, Gonzalez Alfageme A, Saenz Banuelos J. Radiological appearance of diaphragmatic mesothelial cysts. Pediatr Radiol 2003;33(12):855–8.
20. Oyar O, Yesildag A, Gulsoy UK. Bilateral and symmetric diaphragmatic crus lipomas: report of a case. Comput Med Imaging Graph 2002;26(2):135–7.
21. Jacob T, Lescout JM, Bussy E. Malignant diaphragmatic pheochromocytoma. Clin Nucl Med 2002;27(11):807–9.
22. van Rijn AB, van Kralingen KW, Koelma IA. Angioleiomyoma of the diaphragm. Ann Thorac Surg 2000;69(6):1928–9.
23. Kaniklides C, Dimopoulos PA. Diaphragmatic haemangioma. A case report. Acta Radiol 1999;40(3):329–32.
24. Gupta AK, Mitra DK, Berry M. Primary embryonal rhabdomyosarcoma of the diaphragm in a child: case report. Pediatr Radiol 1999;29(11):823–5.
25. Drewes J, Willmann KH. [Primary tumors of the diaphragm] [German]. Thorax 1955;3(1):75–85.
26. Wiener MF, Chou WH. Primary tumors of the diaphragm. Arch Surg 1965;90:143–52.
27. Weksler B, Ginsberg RJ. Tumors of the diaphragm. Chest Surg Clin N Am 1998;8(2):441–7.
28. Mandal AK, Lee H, Salem F. Review of primary tumors of the diaphragm. J Natl Med Assoc 1988;80(2):214–7.
29. Olafsson G, Rausing A, Holen O. Primary tumors of the diaphragm. Chest 1971;59(5):568–70.
30. Akinci D, Akhan O, Ozmen M, et al. Diaphragmatic mesothelial cysts in children: radiologic findings and percutaneous ethanol sclerotherapy. AJR Am J Roentgenol 2005;185(4):873–7.
31. Ueda H, Andoh K, Kusano T, et al. Diaphragmatic cyst with elevated level of serum tissue polypeptide antigen. Thorac Cardiovasc Surg 1992;40(4):195–7.

32. Bugnon PY, Soyez C, Servais B, et al. [Primary non-parasitic cyst of the diaphragm. Review of the literature. Apropos of a case] [in French]. J Chir (Paris) 1988;125(10):582–4.

33. Ruland O, Hoing R, Fiedler C, et al. [Sonographic diagnosis of mesothelial cyst of the diaphragm] [in German]. Ultraschall Med 1987;8(1):51–2.

34. Liou CH, Hsu HH, Hsueh CJ, et al. Imaging findings of intradiaphragmatic bronchogenic cyst: a case report. J Formos Med Assoc 2001;100(10):712–4.

35. Zugel NP, Kox M, Lang RA, et al. Laparoscopic resection of an intradiaphragmatic bronchogenic cyst. JSLS 2008;12(3):318–20.

36. Rozenblit A, Iqbal A, Kaleya R, et al. Case report: intradiaphragmatic bronchogenic cyst. Clin Radiol 1998;53(12):918–20.

37. Oyar O, Kayalioglu G, Cagirici U. Diaphragmatic crus lipoma: a case report. Comput Med Imaging Graph 1998;22(5):421–3.

38. Kalen NA. Lipoma of the diaphragm. Scand J Respir Dis 1970;51(1):28–32.

39. Papachristos IC, Laoutides G, Papaefthimiou O, et al. Gigantic primary lipoma of the diaphragm presenting with respiratory failure. Eur J Cardiothorac Surg 1998;13(5):609–11.

40. Froehner M, Ockert D, Bunk A, et al. Liposarcoma of the diaphragm: CT and sonographic appearances. Abdom Imaging 2001;26(3):300–2.

41. Wolthuis AM, Aelvoet C, Bosteels J, et al. Diaphragmatic endometriosis: diagnosis and surgical management—a case report. Acta Chir Belg 2003; 103(5):519–20.

42. Nezhat C, Seidman DS, Nezhat F, et al. Laparoscopic surgical management of diaphragmatic endometriosis. Fertil Steril 1998;69(6):1048–55.

43. Alifano M, Trisolini R, Cancellieri A, et al. Thoracic endometriosis: current knowledge. Ann Thorac Surg 2006;81(2):761–9.

44. Posniak HV, Keshavarzian A, Jabamoni R. Diaphragmatic endometriosis: CT and MR findings. Gastrointest Radiol 1990;15(4):349–51.

45. Wijnaendts LC, van der Linden JC, van Unnik AJ, et al. Histopathological classification of childhood rhabdomyosarcomas: relationship with clinical parameters and prognosis. Hum Pathol 1994;25(9): 900–7.

46. Raney RB, Anderson JR, Andrassy RJ, et al. Soft-tissue sarcomas of the diaphragm: a report from the Intergroup Rhabdomyosarcoma Study Group from 1972 to 1997. J Pediatr Hematol Oncol 2000; 22(6):510–4.

47. Vade A, Bova D, Borge M, et al. Imaging of primary rhabdomyosarcoma of the diaphragm. Comput Med Imaging Graph 2000;24(5):339–42.

48. Strauch JT, Aleksic I, Schorn B, et al. Leiomyosarcoma of the diaphragm. Ann Thorac Surg 1999;67(4): 1154–5.

49. Cho Y, Hishiyama H, Nakamura Y, et al. A case of leiomyosarcoma of the diaphragm. Ann Thorac Cardiovasc Surg 2001;7(5):297–300.

50. Girard N, Mornex F, Van Houtte P, et al. Thymoma: a focus on current therapeutic management. J Thorac Oncol 2009;4(1):119–26.

51. Mineo TC, Biancari F. Reoperation for recurrent thymoma: experience in seven patients and review of the literature. Ann Chir Gynaecol 1996;85(4):286–91.

52. Rea F, Sartori F, Loy M, et al. Chemotherapy and operation for invasive thymoma. J Thorac Cardiovasc Surg 1993;106(3):543–9.

53. Berruti A, Borasio P, Gerbino A, et al. Primary chemotherapy with adriamycin, cisplatin, vincristine and cyclophosphamide in locally advanced thymomas: a single institution experience. Br J Cancer 1999; 81(5):841–5.

54. Loehrer PJ Sr, Chen M, Kim K, et al. Cisplatin, doxorubicin, and cyclophosphamide plus thoracic radiation therapy for limited-stage unresectable thymoma: an intergroup trial. J Clin Oncol 1997; 15(9):3093–9.

55. Juretzka MM, Horton FR, Abu-Rustum NR, et al. Full-thickness diaphragmatic resection for stage IV ovarian carcinoma using the EndoGIA stapling device followed by diaphragmatic reconstruction using a Gore-tex graft: a case report and review of the literature. Gynecol Oncol 2006;100(3):618–20.

56. dos Santos LA, Modica I, Flores RM, et al. En bloc resection of diaphragm with lung for recurrent ovarian cancer: a case report. Gynecol Oncol 2006;102(3):596–8.

57. Sakakura N, Mori S, Ishiguro F, et al. Subcategorization of resectable non-small cell lung cancer involving neighboring structures. Ann Thorac Surg 2008;86(4):1076–83 [discussion: 1083].

58. Yokoi K, Tsuchiya R, Mori T, et al. Results of surgical treatment of lung cancer involving the diaphragm. J Thorac Cardiovasc Surg 2000;120(4):799–805.

59. Rocco G, Rendina EA, Meroni A, et al. Prognostic factors after surgical treatment of lung cancer invading the diaphragm. Ann Thorac Surg 1999; 68(6):2065–8.

60. Weksler B, Bains M, Burt M, et al. Resection of lung cancer invading the diaphragm. J Thorac Cardiovasc Surg 1997;114(3):500–1.

61. Flores RM, Routledge T, Seshan VE, et al. The impact of lymph node station on survival in 348 patients with surgically resected malignant pleural mesothelioma: implications for revision of the American Joint Committee on cancer staging system. J Thorac Cardiovasc Surg 2008;136(3):605–10.

62. Kent M, Rice D, Flores R. Diagnosis, staging, and surgical treatment of malignant pleural mesothelioma. Curr Treat Options Oncol 2008;9(2–3):158–70.

63. Rathinam S, Venkateswaran R, Rajesh PB, et al. Reconstruction of the chest wall and the diaphragm

using the inverted Y Marlex methylmethacrylate sandwich flap. Eur J Cardiothorac Surg 2004;26(1): 197–201.

64. McConkey MO, Temple CL, McFadden S, et al. Autologous diaphragm reconstruction with the pedicled latissimus dorsi flap. J Surg Oncol 2006;94(3):248–51.

65. Ohsaki Y, Morimoto H, Osanai S, et al. Extensively calcified hemangioma of the diaphragm with increased 99mTc-hydroxymethylene diphosphonate uptake. Intern Med 2000;39(7):576–8.

66. Itakura M, Shiraishi K, Kadosaka T, et al. Chondroma of the diaphragm—report of a case. Endoscopy 1990;22(6):276–8.

67. Chatterjee JS, Powell AP, Chatterjee D. Pleomorphic rhabdomyosarcoma of the diaphragm. J Natl Med Assoc 2005;97(1):95–8.

68. Song HK, Leibold TM, Gal AA, et al. Extraskeletal osteosarcoma of the diaphragm presenting as a chest mass. Ann Thorac Surg 2002;74(2): 565–7.

69. Soysal O, Libshitz HI. Diaphragmatic desmoid tumor. AJR Am J Roentgenol 1996;166(6):1496–7.

70. Tanaka F, Sawada K, Ishida I, et al. Prosthetic replacement of entire left hemidiaphragm in malignant fibrous histiocytoma of the diaphragm. J Thorac Cardiovasc Surg 1982;83(2):278–84.

Reconstructive Techniques After Diaphragm Resection

David J. Finley, MD[a], Nadeem R. Abu-Rustum, MD[b],
Dennis S. Chi, MD[b], Raja Flores, MD[a],*

KEYWORDS
- Diaphragm • Reconstruction • PTFE • Cancer • Resection

Although a rare occurrence, the need for diaphragmatic resection necessitates complete reconstruction to avoid respiratory compromise or the displacement of abdominal contents into the chest. Depending on the extent of resection, the diaphragm can be reconstructed primarily, using synthetic material or autologous tissues. Specific anatomic considerations require a thorough understanding of the diaphragmatic innervation and blood supply to avoid denervation or significant blood loss during resection and reconstruction of the diaphragm.

BASIC ANATOMY

The diaphragm is dome shaped, separating the abdominal compartment from the thoracic cavity, and is the major muscle of respiration. Consisting of muscle fibers that emanate from the chest wall and coalesce at the central tendon, an aponeurosis of fascia fibers, the diaphragm allows vital abdominal structures to remain behind the protection of the lower ribs. The left and right phrenic nerves innervate the diaphragm, entering on the superomedial surface and branch immediately in a radial fashion. The phrenic artery and vein supply most of the blood flow to the diaphragm, although intercostal arterial supply is present along the costal borders, giving the diaphragm a rich blood supply (**Fig. 1**).

The diaphragmatic crus forms the opening for the esophagus, and posterior to this opening is the aorta, passing directly through the muscle fiber decussation. On the right, the inferior vena cava (IVC) and, at times, hepatic veins pass through the diaphragm at the inferior border of the central tendon (between the anterior and right lateral leaves), and they have direct venous communication with the phrenic vein.

INDICATIONS FOR RESECTION

Because primary diaphragmatic tumors are rare, most diaphragm resections are secondary to tumors that invade the diaphragm, including lung cancer, mesothelioma, chest wall tumors, ovarian cancer, and other metastatic lesions. Complete resection of these tumors offers the best chance of survival, necessitating partial and sometimes complete resection of the diaphragm.[1,2]

TYPES OF RESECTION

Depending on the location of the tumor, the type of tumor, and the amount of diaphragm involved, limited resection may be an option. Most tumors require resection with adequate margins, although some require significant margins, such as sarcomas, which often require near complete or complete resection of the diaphragm. Consideration of the location of the tumor is important. Tumors that are peripherally located may require concomitant chest wall resections. Those located medially may involve the phrenic nerve and

[a] Thoracic Service, Department of Surgery, Memorial Sloan-Kettering Cancer Center, 1275 York Avenue, New York, NY 10065, USA
[b] Gynecology Service, Department of Surgery, Memorial Sloan-Kettering Cancer Center, 1275 York Avenue, New York, NY 10065, USA
* Corresponding author.
E-mail address: floresr@mskcc.org (R. Flores).

Thorac Surg Clin 19 (2009) 531–535
doi:10.1016/j.thorsurg.2009.07.007
1547-4127/09/$ – see front matter © 2009 Elsevier Inc. All rights reserved.

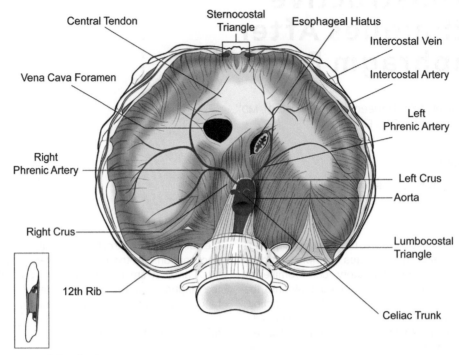

Fig. 1. Anatomy of the diaphragm.

resection can lead to denervation of the diaphragm. This may also require pericardial resection at the same time. These factors must be taken into consideration when planning the best oncologic resection of tumors involving the diaphragm.

Resection of the diaphragm can be performed sharply, using electrocautery or stapling devices. There are not enough data to recommend one technique over the other, but both electrocautery and stapling devices allow for hemostasis during resection. Stapling may provide an added bonus, because the staple line provides a bolster for sutures that might otherwise pull through the diaphragmatic muscle.[3] Keeping the peritoneum intact during resection, as long as it does not involve tumor, may help reduce transdiaphragmatic fluid shifts.

The location of the IVC, hepatic veins, and liver make resection and reconstruction of the right hemidiaphragm more difficult. As the resection progresses, these structures must be identified to reduce the risk of injuring them. Branches of the phrenic vein and artery should also be identified and taken individually to ensure adequate hemostasis before reconstruction. If the phrenic vein is avulsed before adequate exposure of the IVC, the bleeding is difficult to control as it occurs below the diaphragm. Once again, in-depth knowledge of surgical anatomy is necessary for diaphragmatic resection.

TYPES OF RECONSTRUCTION

Most diaphragmatic resections can be repaired primarily, as long as there is adequate tissue that can be brought together without undue tension. A large, nonabsorbable suture should be used in a horizontal mattress fashion to approximate the edges of the defect (**Fig. 2**). Some advocate the use of a second running suture to create a watertight seal to reduce fluid passing between the thoracic and abdominal cavities. In this fashion, defects of up to 8 cm in diameter can be closed. The authors have used a single continuous suture on occasion without any problems.

For a large defect, such as completely resected diaphragm or severely attenuated diaphragmatic tissue, the diaphragm can be reconstructed with synthetic or autologous tissue. Polytetrafluoroethylene (PTFE), 2-mm thick, is an excellent material for reconstructing the diaphragm; it provides the necessary strength and is watertight. The defect in the diaphragm is measured in 2 dimensions, and the PTFE is cut generously to fit the space. For partial resections, the patch is sutured using a running 0 nonabsorbable suture around the edges of the defect, often starting at the medial

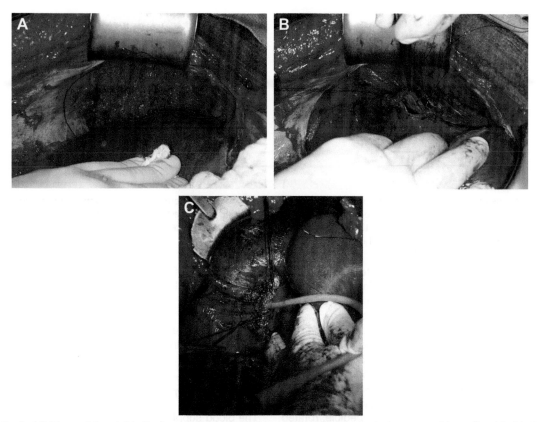

Fig. 2. (*A*) View of the right diaphragm from the abdomen. The diaphragm to be resected is outlined in black (approximately 14 × 6 cm). (*B*) Closure of the defect in the diaphragm, primarily using nonabsorbable suture in an interrupted fashion. Horizontal mattress sutures provide excellent closure and reduce the risk of the stitch tearing through the diaphragmatic fibers. (*C*) Primary repair of the diaphragm near completion. A red rubber catheter is placed in the chest cavity, through the diaphragm to evacuate air before securing the final sutures.

border. The patch is tailored to fit as it is sutured in place, making sure to reduce any laxity in the diaphragm. Care is taken to take full-thickness bites, while avoiding injury to structures below the diaphragm.

For complete diaphragm resections, the patch is measured as described earlier. Starting from the most medial aspect, the PTFE is sutured in place using a running 0 nonabsorbable monofilament suture along the mediastinum, usually to the pericardial edge (**Fig. 3**). Interrupted sutures are then placed around the ribs, following the natural course of the diaphragm from the level of the seventh rib anteriorly to the tenth rib posteriorly to secure the patch in place (**Fig. 4**). Finally, the patch is secured to the posterior crus to anchor it in place (**Fig. 5**). Care must be taken to stretch the patch and place the sutures under some tension to avoid billowing of the patch. The practice of creating a tight patch repair has come into question. Sugarbaker and colleagues[4] reported that with a tight diaphragmatic patch repair, there

was an increased incidence of patch dehiscence compared with the use of a loose 2-patch technique (12% vs 3.8% dehiscence rate, respectively). The 2-patch repair requires 2 pieces of

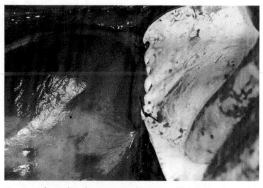

Fig. 3. After diaphragm and pericardial resection, the patch is sutured along the medial border to the pericardium using a running suture. Care is taken not to impede flow through the IVC or hepatic veins.

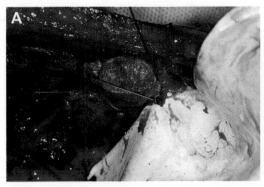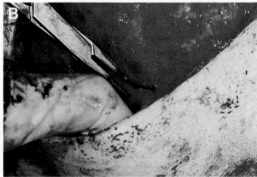

Fig. 4. (*A*) At the level of the costal margin, a stitch is placed around the remnant of the sixth rib to secure the patch in place. (*B*) Stitches are placed around the ribs from outside the chest to allow the patch reconstruction to follow the original contours of the diaphragm. This suture will ultimately be placed through the patch on the inside of the chest and secured on top of the rib.

PTFE, overlapped at the center and stapled together with a thoracoabdominal (TA) stapler. This, in theory, allows the patch to be dynamic, reducing the stress on the sutures.

The latissimus dorsi muscle, as a pedicled flap, can be used to reconstruct the diaphragm.[5,6] Multiple other muscle flaps have also been used, including rectus abdominis, external oblique abdominis, and transversus abdominis muscle flaps, mainly in the pediatric population.[7–9] These flaps are mobilized on a vascular pedicle, rotated into place, and sutured using a large nonabsorbable suture in a running fashion.[6] Using autologous

tissue may be of some benefit in certain situations, especially in children, because the use of synthetic material does not allow for growth as the child ages. It may also be advantageous in patients who are at high risk for infectious complications, including patients with postobstructive pneumonia.

PEARLS AND PITFALLS

The blood supply for the diaphragm is positioned on its inferior surface and often the resection is performed from the chest, making it easy to

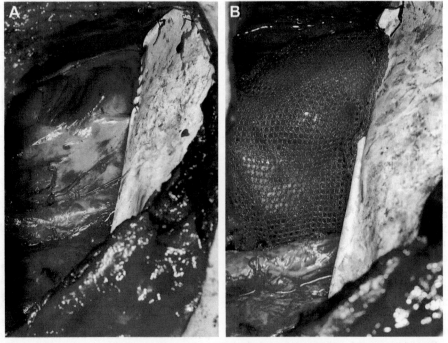

Fig. 5. (*A*) The completed patch repair, without pericardial reconstruction. (*B*) The completed patch repair, with pericardial reconstruction.

transect the phrenic artery and vein before gaining vascular control. Care should be taken to gain control of these vessels along the medial borders of the diaphragm, because they often arise directly from the IVC or aorta and the blood loss can be rapid and significant. The IVC and hepatic veins must also be identified and protected before resection to avoid injuring these 2 structures. Avulsing the phrenic vein from the IVC before adequate exposure can cause profuse bleeding that is difficult to identify and control.

During complete reconstruction of the right diaphragm, care must be taken not to constrict the IVC or hepatic veins along the medial border with the patch. The best way to avoid constricting the IVC or hepatic veins along the medial border is by cutting a notch out of the patch at the level of the IVC. In contrast to this, openings on the left side at the level of the diaphragmatic hiatus should be avoided. During resection of the diaphragm, part of the left crus should be preserved, if possible, and the patch should be secured to the crus to avoid herniation of the stomach, spleen, or other abdominal organs.

The phrenic nerve should be preserved whenever possible, and if injury to the nerve occurs, either by necessity or incidentally, the diaphragm should be plicated to reduce the risk of eventration. Stretching the diaphragm during reconstruction, to remove any redundancy, is essential. This is also true when using autologous tissue, which requires a significant amount of tension to be placed during implantation. If this tenet is not followed, patients will potentially have paradoxic motion of the diaphragm or pathologic elevation, which can lead to respiratory compromise. A tight patch repair with PTFE has been taught historically, although recently this practice has been shown to increase the risk of dehiscence of the patch.[4] Creating a dynamic patch repair may reduce this risk, although this has not been shown in any randomized trials to date.

SUMMARY

Diaphragmatic resection necessitates complete reconstruction to avoid respiratory compromise or the displacement of abdominal contents into the chest. Often the diaphragm can be reconstructed primarily, but with larger or complete resections, reconstruction with synthetic material or autologous tissues is the most appropriate choice. To reduce the risk of denervation of the diaphragm or large intraoperative blood loss, an in-depth knowledge of the diaphragmatic innervation and blood supply are necessary when performing diaphragm resection and reconstruction.

REFERENCES

1. Rocco G, Rendina EA, Meroni A, et al. Prognostic factors after surgical treatment of lung cancer invading the diaphragm. Ann Thorac Surg 1999;68: 2065–8.
2. Weksler B, Bains M, Burt M, et al. Resection of lung cancer invading the diaphragm. J Thorac Cardiovasc Surg 1997;114:500–1.
3. Juretzka MM, Horton FR, Abu-Rustum NR, et al. Full-thickness diaphragmatic resection for stage IV ovarian carcinoma using the EndoGIA stapling device followed by diaphragmatic reconstruction using a Gore-tex graft: a case report and review of the literature. Gynecol Oncol 2006;100:618–20.
4. Sugarbaker DJ, Jaklitsch MT, Bueno R, et al. Prevention, early detection, and management of complications after 328 consecutive extrapleural pneumonectomies. J Thorac Cardiovasc Surg 2004;128:138–46.
5. Bedini AV, Andreani SM, Muscolino G. Latissimus dorsi reverse flap to substitute the diaphragm after extrapleural pneumonectomy. Ann Thorac Surg 2000;69:986–8.
6. McConkey MO, Temple CL, McFadden S, et al. Autologous diaphragm reconstruction with the pedicled latissimus dorsi flap. J Surg Oncol 2006;94:248–51.
7. Hallock GG, Lutz DA. Turnover TRAM flap as a diaphragmatic patch. Ann Plast Surg 2004;52:93–6.
8. Shimamura Y, Gunvén P, Ishii M, et al. Repair of the diaphragm with an external oblique muscle flap. Surg Gynecol Obstet 1989;169:159–60.
9. Simpson JS, Gossage JD. Use of abdominal wall muscle flap in repair of large congenital diaphragmatic hernia. J Pediatr Surg 1971;6:42–4.

Index

Note: Page numbers of article titles are in **boldface** type.

United States Postal Service

Statement of Ownership, Management, and Circulation
(All Periodicals Publications Except Requestor Publications)

1. Publication Title	2. Publication Number	3. Filing Date
Thoracic Surgery Clinics	0 1 3 - 1 2 6	9/15/09

4. Issue Frequency	5. Number of Issues Published Annually	6. Annual Subscription Price
Feb, May, Aug, Nov	4	$242.00

7. Complete Mailing Address of Known Office of Publication (Not printer) (Street, city, county, state, and ZIP+4®)

Elsevier Inc.
360 Park Avenue South
New York, NY 10010-1710

Contact Person
Stephen Bushing

Telephone (Include area code)
215-239-3688

8. Complete Mailing Address of Headquarters or General Business Office of Publisher (Not printer)

Elsevier Inc., 360 Park Avenue South, New York, NY 10010-1710

9. Full Names and Complete Mailing Addresses of Publisher, Editor, and Managing Editor (Do not leave blank)

Publisher (Name and complete mailing address)

John Schrefer, Elsevier, Inc., 1600 John F. Kennedy Blvd. Suite 1800, Philadelphia, PA 19103-2899

Editor (Name and complete mailing address)

Catherine Bewick, Elsevier, Inc., 1600 John F. Kennedy Blvd. Suite 1800, Philadelphia, PA 19103-2899

Managing Editor (Name and complete mailing address)

Catherine Bewick, Elsevier, Inc., 1600 John F. Kennedy Blvd. Suite 1800, Philadelphia, PA 19103-2899

10. Owner (Do not leave blank. If the publication is owned by a corporation, give the name and address of the corporation immediately followed by the names and addresses of all stockholders owning or holding 1 percent or more of the total amount of stock. If not owned by a corporation, give the names and addresses of the individual owners. If owned by a partnership or other unincorporated firm, give its name and address as well as those of each individual owner. If the publication is published by a nonprofit organization, give its name and address.)

Full Name	Complete Mailing Address
Wholly owned subsidiary of	4520 East-West Highway
Reed/Elsevier, US holdings	Bethesda, MD 20814

11. Known Bondholders, Mortgagees, and Other Security Holders Owning or Holding 1 Percent or More of Total Amount of Bonds, Mortgages, or Other Securities. If none, check box. ☐ None

Full Name	Complete Mailing Address
N/A	

12. Tax Status (For completion by nonprofit organizations authorized to mail at nonprofit rates) (Check one)
The purpose, function, and nonprofit status of this organization and the exempt status for federal income tax purposes:
☐ Has Not Changed During Preceding 12 Months
☐ Has Changed During Preceding 12 Months (Publisher must submit explanation of change with this statement)

PS Form 3526, September 2007 (Page 1 of 3) (Instructions Page 3)) PSN 7530-01-000-9931 PRIVACY NOTICE: See our Privacy policy in www.usps.com

---

13. Publication Title		14. Issue Date for Circulation Data Below
Thoracic Surgery Clinics		May 2009

15. Extent and Nature of Circulation			Average No. Copies Each Issue During Preceding 12 Months	No. Copies of Single Issue Published Nearest to Filing Date
a. Total Number of Copies (Net press run)			1550	1300
b. Paid Circulation (By Mail and Outside the Mail)	(1)	Mailed Outside-County Paid Subscriptions Stated on PS Form 3541. (Include paid distribution above nominal rate, advertiser's proof copies, and exchange copies)	662	652
	(2)	Mailed In-County Paid Subscriptions Stated on PS Form 3541 (Include paid distribution above nominal rate, advertiser's proof copies, and exchange copies)		
	(3)	Paid Distribution Outside the Mails Including Sales Through Dealers and Carriers, Street Vendors, Counter Sales, and Other Paid Distribution Outside USPS®	344	311
	(4)	Paid Distribution by Other Classes Mailed Through the USPS (e.g. First-Class Mail®)		
c. Total Paid Distribution (Sum of 15b (1), (2), (3), and (4))		▲	1006	963
d. Free or Nominal Rate Distribution (By Mail and Outside the Mail)	(1)	Free or Nominal Rate Outside-County Copies Included on PS Form 3541	69	53
	(2)	Free or Nominal Rate In-County Copies Included on PS Form 3541		
	(3)	Free or Nominal Rate Copies Mailed at Other Classes Through the USPS (e.g. First-Class Mail)		
	(4)	Free or Nominal Rate Distribution Outside the Mail (Carriers or other means)		
e. Total Free or Nominal Rate Distribution (Sum of 15d (1), (2), (3) and (4))		▲	69	53
f. Total Distribution (Sum of 15c and 15e)		▲	1075	1016
g. Copies not Distributed (See instructions to publishers #4 (page #3))		▲	475	284
h. Total (Sum of 15f and g)		▲	1550	1300
i. Percent Paid (15c divided by 15f times 100)			93.58%	94.78%

16. Publication of Statement of Ownership

☐ If the publication is a general publication, publication of this statement is required. Will be printed in the November 2009 issue of this publication. ☐ Publication not required.

17. Signature and Title of Editor, Publisher, Business Manager, or Owner	Date
Stephen R. Bushing Stephen R. Bushing – Subscription Services Coordinator	September 15, 2009

I certify that all information furnished on this form is true and complete. I understand that anyone who furnishes false or misleading information on this form or who omits material or information requested on the form may be subject to criminal sanctions (including fines and imprisonment) and/or civil sanctions (including civil penalties).

PS Form 3526, September 2007 (Page 2 of 3)

Moving?

Make sure your subscription moves with you!

To notify us of your new address, find your **Clinics Account Number** (located on your mailing label above your name), and contact customer service at:

Email: journalscustomerservice-usa@elsevier.com

800-654-2452 (subscribers in the U.S. & Canada)
314-447-8871 (subscribers outside of the U.S. & Canada)

Fax number: 314-447-8029

Elsevier Health Sciences Division
Subscription Customer Service
3251 Riverport Lane
Maryland Heights, MO 63043